Crack_ed

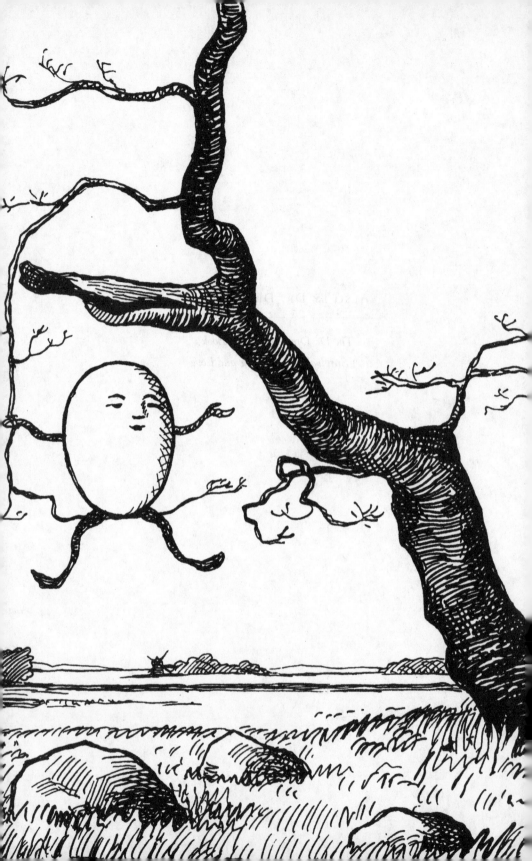

Cracked

PUTTING BROKEN LIVES
TOGETHER AGAIN

A Doctor's Story

DR. Drew Pinsky *with* Todd Gold

10 ReganBooks
Celebrating Ten Bestselling Years
An Imprint of HarperCollinsPublishers

First paperback edition published in 2004.

Designed by Diane Hobbing/Snap Haus Graphics

The Library of Congress has cataloged the hardcover edition as follows:

Pinsky, Drew.
  Cracked : putting broken lives together again: a doctor's story / Drew Pinsky with Todd Gold.
    p. cm.
  ISBN 0-06-009654-3 (hc : alk paper)
  1. Substance abuse—Treatment—Anecdotes. 2. Substance abuse—Patients—Rehabilitation—Anecdotes. 3. Addiction—Services for. 4. Alcoholics—Services for. 5. Substance abuse—Patients—Counseling of. I. Title.

RC564.P56 2003
362.29'18—dc21

2003054817

ISBN 0-06-009655-1 (pbk.)

HB 03.03.2023

For my wife and children

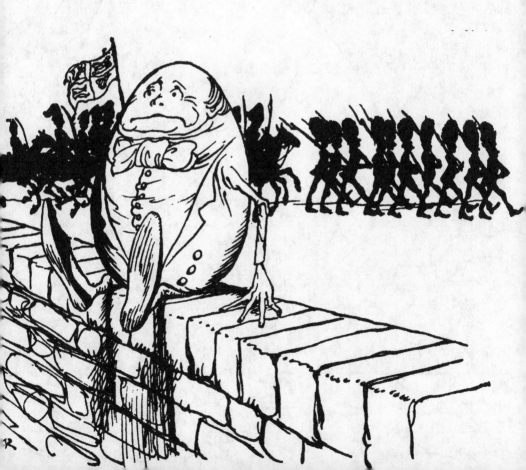

Humpty Dumpty sat on a wall,
Humpty Dumpty had a great fall;
All the king's horses and all the king's men
Couldn't put Humpty Dumpty together again.

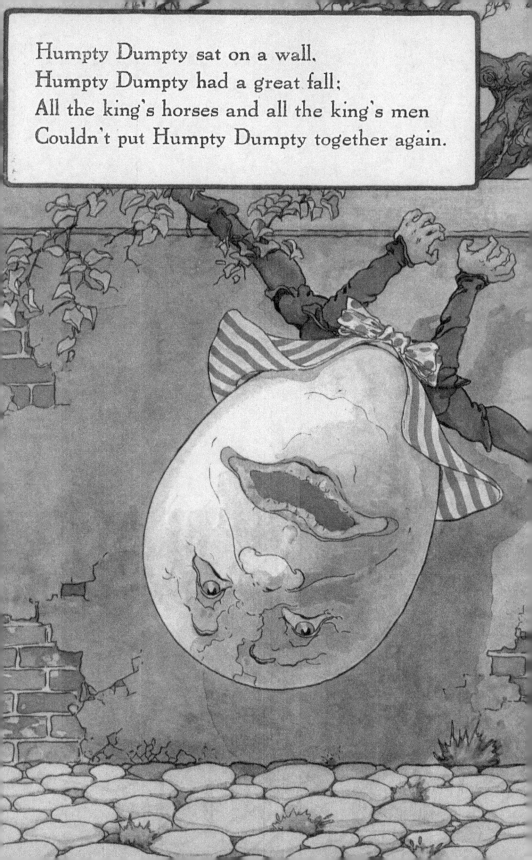

Crack_ed

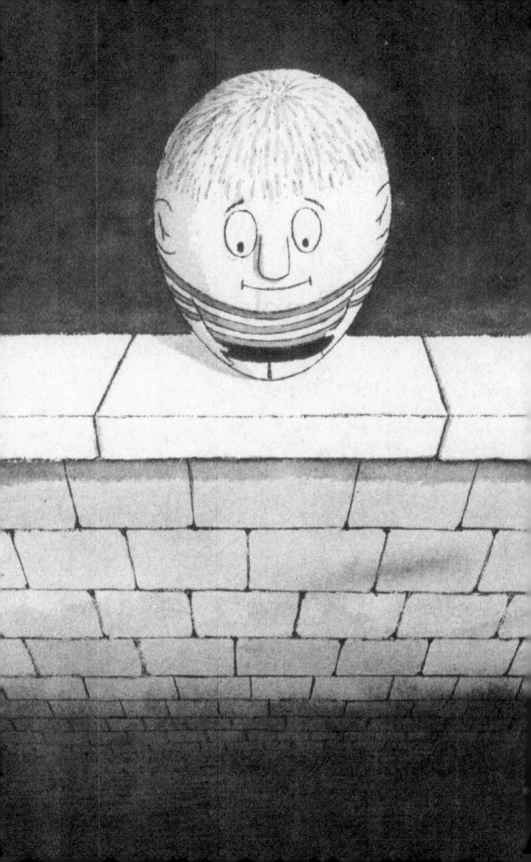

Introduction

FROM THE ROAR of the crowd in the bleachers, I know I've missed something good. It's Sunday afternoon, and I am being torn apart. Actually, I'm tearing myself away from the Little League field, where my ten-year-old sons, Douglas and Jordan, are in a tight spot in the middle of a game. Just a few moments ago I was yelling hitting tips to the boys as my wife, Susan, and my daughter, Paulina, gave me what-are-you-doing-type looks. Then, with Douglas on first and Jordan at bat, my beeper went off. Now I'm headed to the hospital, a medical problem in front of me and a ballgame left behind.

Welcome to my life. Sure, I'm happily married, the father of triplets to whom I'm devoted. But I'm also chief doctor at a chemical dependency unit. So as much as I love watching my sons play ball, and probably could have done so today without risking anyone's life, I know I would've been on my cell phone the whole time—or at least long enough for Susan to say, "Just go."

That's why I'm weaving through traffic, grim-faced, while talking to Kathy, the evening charge nurse. Though she's normally even-tempered and in control, I can hear she's pissed, anxious, and overwhelmed. That alone tells me a lot about the patient: She's a borderline, a trauma survivor, someone who's projecting her pain onto everyone around her, including the nurse.

"It's wild over here," says Kathy, almost chuckling; she realizes she's deflecting the patient's chaos onto me. "Sorry."

"It's okay," I say. "I'm in the car now, though; I can hear you. Run me through it me again."

"I just took in a new patient. She's a twenty-eight-year-old female. Taking thirty to fifty Vicodin a day. Nine milligrams of Ativan. She says that's it. I placed a clonidine patch. She started the narcotic protocol."

"Add in the phenobarb protocol starting at two hundred and forty milligrams. With sixtyQ6 PRN. Routine labs. Pregnancy test if you think it's appropriate. Any IV drug history?"

"No. But I have a problem."

"What's that?" I ask.

"Her mother is here. She's hysterical—she wants to talk to the doctor right away. Like it's not soon enough, if you know what I mean."

"I hope you set some limits with her."

"I tried, but she's really out there. She's beyond wanting to know what's going to happen during treatment. She's major drama."

Indeed she is. When I get to the hospital, I find the woman in mid-flipout. I take her away from her daughter and put her in an empty office. Did I smell alcohol on her breath? Do I have another patient here? She doesn't seem to be impaired, but I wonder if she's going to be a problem later on. I wonder if I should let her drive.

As these and other questions run through my mind, she continues on the attack. "What's going to happen to my baby?" she asks.

"We'll finish detoxing to let her brain settle down so she can begin to think more clearly and engage in the emotional experience of recovery. There are lots of group meetings. She'll get a sponsor. She'll learn how to develop genuine relationships and meaningful connections with other people. And she'll—"

"No, this is not right," she says. "This is typical of how you people have treated my daughter since we arrived. It's all talk, excuses, and explanations. But you saw my baby. Did you see my baby?"

"I did."

"She's in pain. She can barely stand it. No one has said a thing about medication, treatment, maybe physical therapy. We've been here an hour. What are you doing to help her?"

I see more than impatience in this woman's eyes. Feeling abandoned without her daughter to prop her up, she's brought her here under the illusion that treatment will be no different than taking her car into the shop. Unfortunately, she can't just pick her daughter up at four o'clock, overhauled and ready for another five thousand miles. Like most people, this mother doesn't understand what we do. Besides the patients, doctors, and nurses, few people ever get a glimpse of what treatment is really all about. You have to be there, present and involved, because it's not something that can be explained cognitively. It's an experiential process of growth—indeed, of brain change.

"I can't tell you when she'll be better," I say. "Treatment takes time. If I told you anything different, it would be a lie."

But that isn't good enough for her. Midway through my explanation she loses her temper, bursts out of the office, finds her drug-addicted daughter, and drags her down the hall toward the exit. There's chaos and confusion. Everything is crazy for a few moments. "This is all *bull-shit!*" she yells. *"You people don't know what you're doing!"* Then the two of them screech out of the parking lot, leaving Kathy and me standing in front of the unit.

I just shake my head and go back inside.

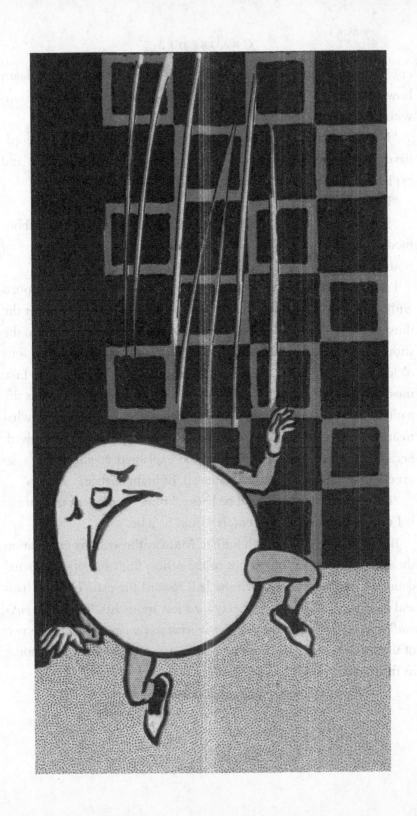

One

IT'S THE SECOND week of a warm August. Early morning. The first one
in my family to rise from bed, I shuffle into the kitchen, start the coffee, and get the newspaper at the end of the driveway. We live in a
ranch-style home perched on the edge of a canyon in the hills above
Pasadena, with deer and coyotes on the prowl, and it's so lovely and
quiet at this hour I might as well be five hundred miles from the harsh-
ness of the city.

The headlines snap me back to reality. I read the *Los Angeles Times*
sports section, sip coffee between box scores, and enjoy the quiet. Soon
my wife, Susan, joins me, followed by the triplets, age ten, who gobble
down breakfast, give us kisses, and go off to summer camp.

Outside, the sun begins its climb into a clear blue sky, and I know
it's going to be, in the words of Randy Newman, "another perfect day"
in L.A.

Perfect for some, perhaps. But not for my patients in the chemical
dependency unit at Las Encinas Hospital, a no-frills, twenty-two–bed

facility popularly known as "rehab." The truth? For many who occupy those beds, it's their last chance before death. To me, it encompasses everything from desperation to the miracle of giving someone a second or third chance at life, at a better life, actually, than they ever dreamed of being able to have.

From the time I back out of my driveway, it takes me twenty minutes to get there. Once I enter the unit, the warm sun is replaced by the low-voltage hum of fluorescent lights. The perfect L.A. day disappears like a song fading from the radio. I step on linoleum, not grass. And when I look up, instead of endless blue sky, I see Ernesto from Operations staring back down at me from inside the ceiling, where he's fixing the air conditioning.

"Good morning, Dr. Pinsky," he says warmly.

"How's it going?" I wave. Then, as I do at the start of each day, I grab my stethoscope, get an opthalmoscope from under the med cart, and pick up the list of patients I need to see.

Today's list is topped by Mark Mitchell, a good-looking thirty-five-year-old in his third day of detox. Mark has been in and out of our care numerous times. His father is a former pro football player turned car dealer, a local celebrity who shows up in gossip columns, has his photographs hanging in restaurants, and seems like a great guy. The truth? He couldn't give a shit about his son. Mark's been hospitalized here at least five times—I can't remember exactly—but he's familiar enough that we've nicknamed him "Mitch." Each time he comes in he looks older, his face creased, grayer beneath his eyes, moving slower.

At the moment, fortunately for me, Mitch isn't as bad as when he was brought in—smelling of vomit and urine, and barely conscious.

But he's still a wreck. Sprawled on his bed—imagine the pieces of a jigsaw puzzle before it's put together—he's tremulous, paranoid, and disorganized. It's normal, all part of the withdrawal from alcohol. The early shift, which admitted Mitch, has already put him on heavy-duty medication to prevent his withdrawal from turning into the DTs, a potentially fatal syndrome where the outflow from the central nervous system is so disorganized that breathing, blood pressure, and other vital functions fail.

Good morning—yeah, right.

Not for Mitch. I stand there for a moment, observing his condition. It takes him several moments to notice I have entered the room. Once he sees me, Mitch jumps to his feet and grabs a piece of paper from the top of his dresser, shoving it toward me as if it were a weapon.

"I'm pissed off," he says angrily, jabbing his finger at a paragraph. "What's this?"

"Wait a minute," I say. "Calm down and let me read."

He's showing me the treatment contract every patient signs on admission. I know what it says without reading it. These are the rules every patient agrees to follow. They include not using drugs, not selling drugs, attending daily group therapy sessions, submitting to urine tests, using the phone only during prescribed hours, and so on. Standard material for someone getting sober. I wrote the contract years ago, and have amended it many times since then. It's nonthreatening to anyone, except those who fear relinquishing control.

Like Mitch. He doesn't know what the hell he's doing or saying. He's out of his mind. His brain is screaming at him to get drunk. Biologically, he craves alcohol more than he wants to breathe. It's driving him crazy. It's hard for him to pay attention to anything else but the urge, and that urge is translated into a scream:

"This is *bogus!* This is *bullshit!* You know it. My cousin is a lawyer, and I know it'll never hold up."

At this rate, I think, neither will he.

I take a deep breath and think of what to say. I could ask if he would like a drink—a vodka tonic? A Heineken? God, that's twisted—though Mitch wouldn't think so. I could try to reason with him, but there's no reasoning with someone this sick. I could call his cousin and threaten to countersue. (Good thing I'm not a lawyer.) I could slap him across the face, the way they used to do in Three Stooges movies, and hope it startles him into sanity. Or I could just listen and nod.

Actually, my fantasy would be to zap him with something—a laying-on of hands, a magic shot or electric shock—and have him all better, sober, clean, with no desire to drink again. That's *my* sickness. I want to rescue everyone. I don't need to turn water into wine or walk on water, but healing the sick would be dandy. Better still, I'd like everyone to be okay. I'd like to stop the suffering and discomfort in the world. Not too much to ask, right?

But that's what makes *me* feel good.

I'm a realist, though. Mitch is more adversarial than most patients, but he's hardly the worst of those making their temporary home at Las Encinas. The unit is a single-story bungalow. It's part of an old-fashioned psychiatric hospital, on thirty rolling acres, that was used many times as a backdrop in old Hollywood movies. Stars from the golden era came here to dry out. W. C. Fields actually died here.

Las Encinas isn't posh enough to make *People* magazine, though. It doesn't have ocean views, like the rehabs catering to the current crop of troubled celebrities. Neither does it have any Oscar contenders. My patients tend to be more like Mitch than like Robert Downey Jr., though we do admit individuals representing every possible facet of society, from the rich to the destitute to the socially prominent to the disconnected.

What do they have in common?

Heroin. Cocaine. Vicodin. Crystal meth. Alcohol. Klonopin. Pot. Combinations of all of the above.

They're addicts.

They're desperate.

They're in retreat from the world.

They're brought by spouses, parents, friends, or ambulances.

Each one has a different story, but they all arrive for the same basic reason: Their lives are out of control.

Mitch was brought two mornings earlier by paramedics from a nearby hospital after he'd been found in a semiconscious, delirious state in an alley behind a bar. He has no idea how close he came to dying.

"Do you know why you're here?" I ask.

After a second or two of staring at me blankly, he picks up a pencil and scribbles a note on the back of his contract. Then he hands it to me.

It says, "Who are you?"

I don't have the time for this. Nor do I like this guy much. But I'm willing to play along. I take out my pen.

"I am Dr. Pinsky," I write.

Some part of him knows this. He allows me to examine him. I listen to his heart and lungs. It's a cursory checkup, takes a minute or two. Some patients draw you in; others have the opposite effect. As he gets through withdrawal, Mitch can be downright charming—I know this from previous stays. He treats the staff with the familiarity of a regular. At the moment, though, he's anything but approachable. My challenge, as well as the staff's, is to stay emotionally attuned without getting overtaken by the intensity of his needs and emotions.

Challenge Number 1: Get him to begin managing his urges.

"I want you to start going to group," I say.

He writes another note and hands it to me.

It says, "And I want you to go to hell."

Instead I go to Room 421—which, as it turns out, might be the same thing.

The room is occupied by a new patient described to me by the charge nurse, Alexi, as "a total mess."

Alexi is the field general among the nurses, attendants, and counselors who comprise the unit's staff. Most of the staff works in the daytime; only a few nurses remain at night. All are highly skilled, insightful, dedicated individuals with a range of experience that gives them unique perspective into the patients. Some of the counselors are former patients. Others have done this type of work longer than I have. Our patients are manipulative, secretive, frightened, paranoid, and unstable, but very few things happen on the floor without one of our team of staffers being aware of it.

Alexi is the best of them all. As the charge nurse, she supervises everything that happens in the unit from admissions to discharge. She is the Radar O'Reilly of our MASH unit: knowledgeable, levelheaded, firm, unflappable, with a great sense of humor. Aside from being a great nurse, she has an uncanny ability to anticipate everything that happens here, and knows exactly how to react.

When I arrived earlier today, Alexi was bent over the counter at the nursing station, filling out a form while people waited. Too busy to say hello, she kicked up her leg in back and wiggled her foot at me. I was supposed to understand, and I did.

She's indispensable. Now in her early forties, Alexi grew up in Yugoslavia during what she calls, acerbically, the Golden Age of Communism. She emigrated to the United States after marrying her scientist husband just after she turned twenty-one. They have one pre-teen daughter. She abhors women who have more than one child. "Breeders," she scoffs. "I'd kill myself before I stayed home with three kids and drove an SUV." She regularly complains that American culture has made kids way too soft. Sometimes she jokes that we should have boot camps instead of rehabs.

"There may be more sophisticated approaches," I tell her.

"I know, I know," she says. "Of course, if we just had plain old alcoholics, I'm telling you the boot camps would work."

"Maybe."

Today's theme?

"Last night I got home and told my daughter to pick up a broom and hold it while she watched her television shows," she says.

"Why?" I ask.

"She needs to get used to it. I told her she'll be doing that if she doesn't work harder at school," she says.

Alexi loves the work as much as I do. On our way to Room 421, she gives me a rundown on the patient.

"What a mess this one is. She's on cocaine, Oxycontin, pot, Klonopin, and maybe—"

"A real Girl Scout," I interrupt.

"She's going to be a handful. She's totally borderline." Then she pauses. "She's so *cute*."

Bingo.

If Alexi likes a patient, I've learned by now to get out the hammer and nails and board up the windows. She's never met a drug-addicted sociopath she didn't adore. It's not that she loves down-and-out dirt-balls. Rather, she's entertained by the drama of the borderlines, the charm and charisma of the sociopaths.

Giggling, she covers her mouth, embarrassed by her own co-dependency shining through.

We hear screams from inside the room.

Alexi's eyes light up. "See. Doesn't she sound funny, all that carrying on?"

A moment later I'm staring at the patient—at least the little bit of her I can see clearly. She's curled up on the floor in the far corner beside the bed. She reminds me of an animal trying to hide. Frightened, suffering pain, a biological mess, Amber lets us guide her into the bed. She quickly pulls the covers up to her chin, shaking and crying. It's been about ten hours since she passed out. Her husband brought her into the hospital, then left for work. From what I see in these first few minutes, I'd say she's fortunate to be alive.

"It's impossible to tell what she's really been doing," says Alexi. "At first, she said she was taking fifteen Oxycontin a day. But then she changed her story—it was two a day. And then it was thirty, sometimes. She also said something about eight hundred milligrams of Valium."

"Any IV drug use?" I ask.

"Hard to say. She denied it at first, but then she said she'd been doing speed. She doesn't have any tracks."

I make a fist, put it to my mouth, and blow on my hand in frustration.

At this point only Amber knows the intimate details of her use, the truth about the years of ugliness that have paved her road here. But I've seen enough young women like her to know what I'm dealing with, and it tears at my gut to confront this over and over again.

Amber is twenty-six, with a model's lissome figure and dark coloring. Her father, I learn, was a terror who left her mother but periodically returned to harass his ex-wife and daughter. There are the first hot buttons of trauma—abandonment, helplessness, the rupture of attachment with someone they love and idealize. Amber's relationships have been similarly chaotic. She has continued to be exploited by men, including her husband, whom I haven't met and to be perfectly truthful might not want to. Her looks have always given her trouble. I start to say something profound about the burden of having perfect looks in our culture, but then I stop myself. It's redundant. I see the twisted consequences in front of me.

"When did this all start for you?" I ask.

"What do you mean?" she says.

"When did you start smoking pot?" I ask, knowing marijuana or alcohol would have been her first drugs.

"Twelve."

"Did you smoke every day?"

"No."

"Every other day?"

"Well . . ."

"How about five out of seven?"

"Yeah, I guess."

First encounters like this are interesting. There's a big, powerful dynamic at work in the room. Though she lets me ask about her medical and drug history, it's not clear at this point that Amber even wants to get better. The only thing she really wants from me right now is relief—which means drugs. She wants a prescription. Not a relationship, not a savior. I'm just standing in her way, unless I can provide her with medication. To her, I'm a capsule on legs.

Of course I would never fully admit that to myself. To acknowledge not existing in her eyes would be too painful for me. I *have* to matter. Why? Because to me, witnessing the collapse of those who were abused and molested as children is almost too much to bear. The emotional fallout is profound. In a way, it's part of my own pathology; I feel the presence of the developmentally arrested traumatized child within patients like Amber, and I let that child invade me. I need to help her so that both of us can feel better.

"When was the last time you used?" I ask.

Amber bites her lip and grimaces.

"It hurts so bad," she says. "Can you just put me to sleep?"

I turn to Alexi for the answer.

"She said she hasn't used since last night, but I think she's got something on board now. Her belongings were clean. If you ask me, though, she still seems loaded."

I agree.

As that wears off, Amber will feel even worse.

"She's going to be detoxing soon, so have the med nurse get a clonidine TTS-3 patch on her right now," I say. "You can also give her Neurontin four hundred milligrams QID, since we really don't know how much benzodiazepine she's been exposed to. No doubt she's going to need a loading dose of phenobarbital. Let's also give her the usual Robaxin, Bentyl, and Motrin per the protocol. Then call the lab and order an HIV and hepatitis screen on the blood they drew this morning. Make sure we get a pregnancy test, too."

We spend a little more time with her, but there's not much else to do except step back and wait for a moment during her withdrawal when we can let her know that we can help her feel better, as long as she listens and does what we say. That moment is clearly not now. Amber is locked in a biological prison. She's so neurobiologically impaired that her responses to our requests are meaningless. Later, she won't remember them anyway.

She clutches a little worn-out teddy bear she's brought from home. The bear is missing an eye and part of an ear, I notice, and its fur has been picked bare in spots, but the red stitching at the mouth still forms a cute smile. I pray that Amber will hold up as well.

But I don't know. Right now she's gripped by pain and fear, and without any of her usual escapes, she yells and moans in agony.

"It's going to get worse," I say. "It's going to be miserable. But we're going to make it tolerable."

"Can I have something right now?"

"Alexi's on it."

When Alexi and I are in the hall, she starts to giggle again.

"I told you she was something," Alexi says.

"Yup, we're going to be in for it," I say. "I hope she'll stick around long enough to wake up and want to get better." But I don't know.

A moment later, I'm down the hall when Amber screams. *"Alexi! I can't take this! Get in here. I need something!"*

"What the hell is that?" asks Dr. Peter Finley, the unit's program director.

Finley, a stocky man with curly black hair, a moustache, and glasses, is basically my counterpart. Whereas I manage the medical care, he handles the psychological. Together, we make sure the patient gets what he or she needs during treatment. Finley has an amazing grasp of the psychological syndromes that affect addicts; he also has exceptional judgment—and there are lots of doctors with great knowledge and shitty judgment. On top of all this he's a first-class storyteller, with a tale for every situation.

"She's a new patient," I say, referring to Amber's plea for help.

"Makes me think of a woman I worked for when I was an assistant at an insurance company during college," he says. "I'll have to tell you about that sometime. But you need to deal with the woman in three-oh-two."

He doesn't need to say much more. The woman in 302, an opiate addict in her late thirties with a difficult personality disorder, has been horrible lately. For the past week, she's driven the staff crazy with her constant demands. She lies and manipulates, and when that's not enough she yells and lashes out.

"She's a pain in the ass," I say.

"We'll just have to build a better cage," says Finley, and launches into the story of one of his dogs that kept escaping until he finally constructed a better fence around his backyard.

I go into 302. Her name is Katherine, and she's been acting like a member of the British royal family, ordering staff around and insisting on a variety of privileges—particularly unrestricted use of her cell phone. We allow phone calls between 7:00 and 10:00 P.M., but she has been demanding unrestricted calling privileges because, as she has told everyone within earshot, her nine-year-old son, the youngest of her three children, is chronically ill. According to her, he's liable to die at any minute.

"So is she," Alexi mutters under her breath every time.

I suspect Katherine has been calling dealers, though she hasn't tested positive—at least not yet.

Katherine is one of those personality types who make you feel their awful feelings right along with them. She gets under your skin. That's a good way to spot a borderline: They defend against their own miserable feelings by projecting them onto other people. Trouble is, I'm a perfect receptacle. I don't need her feelings on top of my own.

None of us do.

I want Katherine off the phone and complying with the rules. As a compromise, I suggest keeping her phone at the nursing station. If it rings, I tell her, we'll get her immediately. That's impossible, she says, angry and dismissive. So I clamp down entirely. If the rules aren't followed to the letter, I tell her, she will get kicked out. After digesting the consequences, she barrages me with all kinds of crazy excuses, accusing me of being cruel and unfair.

"My child is going to die," she says. "He's connected to tubes. They get badly infected. You're a doctor. What about that don't you understand?"

"What is it about checking in between seven and ten that's so unreasonable?" I respond. "If there's a problem at another time, we'll get you."

"My husband and children live back East. Isn't it enough I'm out here? With the time difference, I'll wake everyone up. It'll be the middle of the night."

I stand my ground, but that only encourages her to act like an animal beating against a cage. At the same time, though, I know I can't ignore the issue of her son. After giving it some thought, I telephone her husband (which I should've done long before, of course) and ask about their son's condition. Turns out the boy hasn't had a health problem in four years. He is, her husband tells me, perfectly stable.

"And his lines?" I ask.

"Not a problem. We haven't had an emergency since I can remember."

My decision about the phone will stand: Katherine will have to deal with containment, and she'll likely do better for it. Borderlines challenge boundaries, but they actually feel safer when they're held. Precisely like little children.

In the meantime, as Katherine and I talk, I take a fresh look at her. What's really going on inside her?

This is a woman who's just transferred from another hospital after going through a rapid opiate detox, a highly controversial procedure in which the system is flooded with medication that blocks the body's receptors for opiates and induces a profound state of withdrawal. The detox so profound it could kill a person if she weren't held under general anesthesia for about eight hours.

The people promoting such treatment believe they're accelerating a withdrawal that would normally take a week or two into a convenient eight hours. *Hooked on heroin? Popping 40 Vicodin a day? Don't worry. You can schedule your withdrawal between business appointments.* Don't believe it. The very idea betrays the fundamental misunderstanding most people share—mistaking detox for treatment.

Katherine is a perfect example of a user who thinks all she needs to do is get off the drugs. Getting off is the necessary first step, of course. It's dramatic, and interesting. But it's only the first step in treating the disease. It's like getting into position to do the work.

Katherine is falling apart all over the place. Having hid the truth about what she'd been using—a common tactic among addicts—now, in addition to her opiate withdrawal, she's dealing with a Valium habit, too. She's a mess in every way. She has discovered that there aren't any quick fixes.How can there be, when the patient has used drugs to regulate emotions she can't manage normally? Generally, these overwhelming emotions are related to childhood traumas—pain, abuse, neglect, abandonment, and overall feelings of powerlessness. There aren't any simple eight-hour cures for that.

I don't go all the way into Katherine's room. You don't want to mess with a dangerous angry borderline—that anger is too easily projected directly onto you. Everything becomes your fault; filled with hostility, they're liable to start accusing you of things, from simple neglect to sexual misconduct.

So I stand in the doorway. Seeing me alone with a dangerous patient, Alexi stops and stands behind me.

"We made a decision. There will be no phone," I say with finality.

The stake has been put in the ground.

I feel a tightening in my stomach, preparing for Katherine's angry onslaught, and I get it. She comes at me from a completely different direction. "Have you called my *real* doctor, Dr. Smith, who did my detox?" she says, her jaw so tight it barely moves. "He told me I would get much more medication than you're giving me."

She's attacking me personally.

"I will certainly notify Dr. Smith of our treatment plan once we get to know you better. Right now you're getting enough medication to detox safely."

No way around it—Katherine is going to take us for a ride. I can't predict where that might end up. "Jesus Christ," I say to Alexi and several of the counseling staff at the nursing station. "We have so many sick patients. Do you think anyone here is interested in recovery?" My job is to evaluate these people at the beginning of their journey, and to be honest, the success rate is mixed. It's easy to get frustrated by patients. They don't follow directions. They're paranoid and distrustful. They see me as a drugstore, if they acknowledge me at all.

"I have a patient who just presented a courageous first step this morning in my group," one counselor says.

"That patient of mine, Joan Bayturn, went to Sober Living," another adds.

"So there's some recovery going on?" I ask. "You mean we're actually having an effect here?"

I know we help. At times it just gets hard to see it.

Some days the beds at Las Encinas are filled with somatically preoccupied heroin addicts, there because their families dragged them in. They aren't the least bit interested in getting better. They're usually manipulative, angry, and hostile. Those are times that try even the unit's most dedicated staffers. Other days I find the biological effects of drugs playing out in the brains of my patients in interesting, not always predictable ways. When these people are also motivated, I can sometimes have the almost spiritual experience of helping return near-dead human beings to life.

If I get angry, it's at the bigger picture. In general, our culture offers us solutions that only intensify our problems. I'm prone to rant about this, I know—but after all, surgeons are permitted to rage against cigarettes and fatty foods, psychologists about poor communication skills. So why shouldn't I go off on the culture?

I have plenty of reasons to call the culture up on charges. Katherine. Amber. Mitch. And hundreds more just like them. The culture is like a living, breathing beast that feeds its own need to exist and grow at the expense of the individual. Our world is full of people with narcissistic problems who look to escape those feelings and be gratified—and the culture steps right up to meet those needs. Many of those contributing to the culture are sick themselves. It doesn't take a shrink to count the number of celebrities who end up in rehab, getting into fights, or posing for mug shots. The media has become an instant-response machine, ratcheting our tolerance ever upward in cycles of arousal and gratification. All of this can be arresting, fun, sexy; most of all, it sells. But it doesn't heal.

What our culture lacks are honest messages about what it really means to be a healthy human being. Or how you make humans grow. These are sort-of-boring topics that won't sell Budweiser or Nikes. Cervantes, writing in *Don Quixote,* goes on a rant like this about theater of the early 1600s. He has the same complaint. Just because people gravitate to something doesn't make it good or right. I want more messages about how healthy humans are created, and as much as I want them, others need them.

Amber is laying on her bed when I see her again. A few hours have passed since I saw her last. Her room is still as dark as she can make it. She also has the heat turned uncomfortably high, to counter the chilling effect of opiate withdrawal. Even so, she still complains about being cold.

I look at her chart again. She's twenty-six, married to an older man, and employed as a receptionist at an advertising company in Hollywood.

What's the longest she's been clean? I don't know.

Does she want to get sober? I don't know that either.

What I do know for sure is that Amber has begun to detox. In simple terms, she's in utter hell. She is sick and getting sicker. Why? Her body is in a state of hyperstimulation, her nervous system overwhelmed and reacting to every little sensation. If not for the central nervous system depressants we've given her, Amber would be screaming for us to put her out of her misery.

She might do that anyway. It goes with the territory.

I pull a chair up next to her bed and sit down. I want to give her some reassurance, establish rapport, and check on the alchemy of what we're doing. Amber looks at me from a thousand miles away. All I see is a young woman in misery. She's craving drugs, and that deeply physical craving hurts worse than a normal healthy human being can imagine.

"Help me," she says.

I know what that means. "We're giving you everything you can safely take," I say.

"I need something now." She moans. "It hurts so badly."

I believe her, but I sit there unmoved. I'm not being callous. This sort of pain is just part of the process of withdrawal. It's a necessary evil. But it's surface stuff. Eventually it goes away. The difficult part is the unexpressed pain that's buried far beneath the surface, the original hurt around which everything else is structured.

I fish around for something positive. Though it might not appear so, she is doing better. She's calmer, and that calms me down.

"Why are you here?" I ask. It's my standard opening line. "You've been doing this for years. Why are you here today?"

The purpose is to find out the source of the patient's motivation to get sober. The initial response, I know, will be some obfuscating bullshit. No one ever comes right out and says, "The court sent me." Nor do they say, "I lost my job and my girlfriend is leaving me." Eventually we get to that. For the most part, they say, "I just got tired of living like this." Which is true. But they've been tired of it for a long time. I want to know why *today*. What got you here at this moment?

Sometimes they have to think about it. Even when the court actually did send them.

Other times, I have to dig for it.

I don't know why it's so hard for patients to give me a real answer. Amber is typical. "I don't know why I'm here," she says.

"You don't know?"

She rolls her eyes and lets me know she has no patience for this.

"Okay. I can't keep living like this. I'm sick of being sick."

Nice try. She's heard that line before, and maybe before it's worked. But I let it sit there. I want something honest.

"I can't go on like this," she continues. "I got a DUI. My husband is pissed at me. I'm tried of all the crap."

"There we go," I say. "Keep going. Drugs have been ruining your life for a long time. I imagine your husband didn't all of a sudden get pissed off for the first time. Why are in you treatment *now?*"

"I told you," she says faintly. "I can't go on like this."

"But why today? I've never met an addict who woke up one day and decided to get sober. It doesn't happen like that. There has to be a whole lot of shit coming down for you to want to stop. What happened?"

"My family has had it with me," she says, dragging a tear across her cheek with the back of her hand. "If I don't get it together this time, I'm going to end up on the street. I know it. They're fed up with me. It's like, either I get help or they're out." She suddenly winces. "Can't you give me something?"

Not now.

Despite her discomfort, Amber complies when I tell her to lay back so I can give her a cursory physical. Like anyone in her condition, she complains of extreme pain. But discomfort may be a closer description of what she's feeling. She is agitated, craving, feeling like she wants to jump out of her skin. Every place on her body hurts—her joints, her muscles, her arms and legs, her back and neck especially. If I could see her brain, it would be throbbing, too.

That's withdrawal.

All in all, though, Amber is in fair shape. Her youth gives her some resiliency. It has also provided her with a few tattoos; several piercings, including one to the side of her nose; and a few strands of blue and red highlights in her otherwise brown hair. She is a very pretty girl. I think Truman Capote once said something like, Beauty makes its own rules. I might add from experience that beauty also suffers its own tragedies. From Marilyn Monroe to the various Hollywood stars I've treated, I wonder why is it that so many beautiful young women suffer. There's no reason Amber has to be another tragedy.

"Am I going to die?" she asks.

"No," I say.

"I feel like it."

"Yeah, I'm sure you do. It's got to be awful. But we're going to get through this. We're going to help you."

I leave the room. She's given me a few positive morsels. Katherine has been a bummer, but I have hope for Amber. I want to have hope.

I ask Alexi if I'm needed for anything else.

"Go," she says. "Get out of here."

I take a step and then stop and turn back to her. I have a last-minute feeling to get rid of before going home.

"You know something? I hate the feeling I get from patients like Amber. I'm trying to help, but she looks at me like I'm a perpetrator. Just one more person in her life who's going to take advantage, abuse, or let her down."

"You have to start building from somewhere," says Alexi. "How much is she complaining?"

"She really wants some more meds," I say.

"She asked every minute or so?"

"She insisted something was wrong with her back or her neck. But I examined her, and it's just the withdrawal. God knows how long she's been numbing and neglecting her central nervous system with drugs, and now it's crackling like an exposed wire."

"Luckily for us, it's just the start." Alexi smiles. "I have a feeling about this one."

"Good or bad?"

"Just a feeling. Let's see how she is in a few days."

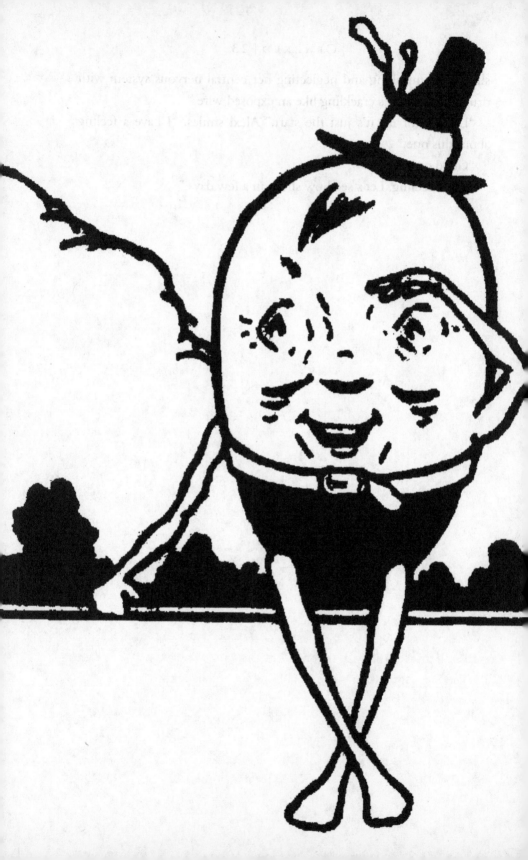

TWO

AFTER A TWO-day absence from the unit, I'm greeted at the nursing station by a very busy and preoccupied Yugoslavian. I feel as if I'm interrupting her in the middle of something more important.

"Angry?" I ask.

"What are you talking about?" she says. "I'm busy."

"Frustrated? Come on. I sense it."

Alexi handles a lot of work, aggravation, and complaining, and she does much of it thanklessly. Not that she's looking for thanks for her everyday work—making sure that everyone is going to group, that detoxes are going as they should, that paperwork is completed. She does all that for many of the same reasons I do. We have to. We're compelled by a force that we probably don't understand as clearly as we should.

Alexi isn't prone to dramatizing her frustration, but this time I can tell she needs to release some of her frustration. She's turned inward; she doesn't want to trade idle conversation the way we usually do at the start of the day. I take a seat on the counter, roll up my sleeves, and let her know that I'm ready to listen.

She starts with Mark.

"How bad did he get?" I ask.

It's not him, she says. He was his usual self. After his encounter with me, he made it to his first group. The next day, as he woke up a bit more, he took it over.

"Mr. Know-It-All," she says, rolling her eyes, bored.

"As he always is," I say.

"Holding court," Alexi says. "He told all the other patients about their problems and what they needed to do."

"He's so program-savvy. He's knows it all cognitively, like he's memorized a part in a play. But emotionally he hasn't grasped a thing. He's never addressed his own issues."

"Not only that," Alexi says. "Last night he left."

"He did what?"

"He checked himself out, muttering something about everyone being full of shit."

"That's the pot calling the kettle black, isn't it?"

"Usually he stays longer," Alexi says. "For some reason, though, it really bothered me this time. I'm worried, because he seemed sicker."

"I'm sure we haven't seen the last of him."

I try to lighten her mood, joking around with her a bit, but after a minute or two she waves her hand, telling me *enough*.

Time for the next problem—Amber.

"You wouldn't believe that one," she says. "Dr. Bloom had to completely snow her with phenobarbital. She was absolutely bouncing off the walls. Carrying on like that. Screaming, crying, throwing herself around the unit. She got all the other patients involved in her drama."

"How's she this morning?"

"She's better today. But only because she's still out of it."

"Let's get a look at her."

As we head to her room, I'm a half-step ahead of Alexi, who is still relaying the highlights of Amber's antics. She was at the med window, demanding more pills, falling all over herself when the nurses said no, growing more and more desperate. Predictable, I think.

We get to Amber's room, listen for something to clue us into what we are in for, and trade a look that says, "Okay, here it comes."

Inside, Amber is curled up on her bed, dressed in blue jeans and a T-shirt. It's dark inside. The curtains are drawn, preventing sunlight from entering. It might as well be nighttime. It *is* for Amber, anyway; unable to venture beyond the cocoon of her painful detox, she's trying to hide out from the stimuli of the outside world.

She makes eye contact as soon as we enter, turning on her side as if inviting conversation.

"How are you today?" I ask softly.

"Not good," she says, as if she's talking in slow motion. "Alexi won't give me anything for the pain."

Alexi interjects, "She's getting all her PRNs."

For the first time Amber looks directly into my eyes, with such clarity I can't miss it: She's trying to make a connection.

"I don't know why you won't give me more," she says. "Nobody believes the pain I'm in. If you believed me, you'd give me more meds."

"Pain is a normal part of withdrawal," I say. "It will end soon."

And then maybe she'll turn down the frigging heat in the room. It feels like the Mojave in here. But of course I don't say anything about that.

"We're giving you everything we can possibly, safely give you," I add, which is something I find myself saying to patients all day long.

Amber couldn't care less. She's already past me, and on to her next tactic. There is almost a coquettishness to her body language, a slight curve to her back as she lays on the bed, her chest arching ever so openly, which I understand is the way someone like Amber is accustomed to dealing with men. I read the invitation—and feel invaded by her. It is scary and uncomfortable as I feel my body reacting, and I think, *I have to put a stop to this. Get going,* I tell myself. *Get to business.*

Quickly, I listen to her heart and chest, making sure nothing medical is going on. She is okay. I give Alexi a look that says, "Let's go."

In retrospect, I have missed an opportunity for tuning more into the painful source of her behavior. But I could not get past the way she made me feel.

Out in the hall, Alexi cracks up. "You better be careful of that one," she says.

"What do you mean?"

"Oh my God!" Alexi laughs. "Did you see how she looked at you?"

I did, but I'm not admitting it. Neither am I finding the situation as funny as Alexi is. I stick to business.

"She's clearly oversedated from all the phenobarb," I say. "In fact, the medicine only seems to be escalating her. Let's taper her off and then see what we've got. Only give her the PRN phenobarbital. Decrease the Neurontin to one hundred milligrams TID for three days, and then stop. Push the alpha 2 agents if you see any objective signs of opiate withdrawal."

Alexi nods.

"One more thing," I add. "Stop looking at that Victoria's Secret catalog I saw on your desk. It's clouding your judgment."

I have a better rapport with Debra, a twenty-eight-year-old working in marketing at one of the television networks. She is preppie-style pretty. Slender. Short brown hair. Tiny glasses that probably cost $350. I picture her five years earlier as a bookish partier at an East Coast college like Sarah Lawrence or Wesleyan.

Debra has made a good impression on the staff. Aside from a trendy

Fred Segal wardrobe—she dresses stylishly rather than provocatively—
she is earnest, insightful, bright, and polite, which goes a long way
among a staff used to belligerence and difficulty. I notice she is writing
diligently in a journal. Seeing me, she looks up and says she is working
on the first of AA's twelve steps, admitting her powerlessness over
drugs and the way it's made her life unmanageable.

"I caught you on *GMA*," she says.

"And?"

"You're great. Mr. Media. I never watch *GMA*, but I'm boycotting
the *Today* show until Matt Lauer's hair grows back."

"How are you doing?"

"Uh," she says, shrugging. Then she turns serious. "I'm jonesing for
my BlackBerry."

Missing a small computer should be her biggest problem. Debra is
in her third week as a patient. For the first ten days, she went through
utter hell withdrawing from Soma, a muscle relaxer the liver converts
into the old-fashioned Miltown. She also suffered from akathesia, an
extreme agitation that caused her to constantly pace and rock, wring-
ing her hands and rubbing her arms in response to a vague pain.
Unable to recall all but the last of those miserable days, Debra simply
knows she doesn't want to go through any of that ever again.

"You're so much better," I say. "I'm so pleased."

She shakes her head.

"Words don't even describe what I went through," she says.

Indeed. But there was more. A few days earlier, she'd been talking
to another patient in the lounge. This guy, whose name was Harold,
was asking about her childhood. It began as a normal conversation; he
was interested in her. But in the course of answering, Debra revealed
that her brother had sexually abused her as a child. She had never spoken about the incident before. As she revealed this, Harold, in his
desire to help, pushed her to confess more and more details.

All of a sudden Debra was in the position of a victim needing rescue, and Harold was ready to oblige. It made him feel worthwhile to be her rescuer, but it left Debra helpless again, powerless and frightened. She needed to learn to manage her feelings on her own.

Instead she was seized by a full-blown post-traumatic stress attack. Heated up by the biology of her withdrawal, she collapsed in a ball, crying and gasping for air.

Fortunately, Alexi and I had been right there for her. We were present and calm. We talked her through it. She got better.

Later, I explained what had happened, and advised her that she shouldn't try to deal with all that trauma until she was in a more solid biological state and more secure. Don't worry about it, I advised. First she needed to get detoxed, and then to start working on her ability to attach to people and reconnect with the world—everything that drugs allowed her to avoid.

Once she was further along in recovery, she could start to deal with the fallout of this long-ago trauma.

"You mean I'm going to have to get into this someday?" she asked.

"We don't believe anymore that you have to reexperience the trauma," I say, struggling to put complicated new theory into a few simple words. "The trauma left you feeling you couldn't trust people. As a result, you never learned how to use interpersonal connection to help you regulate your feelings. That's what you'll develop over time."

"Okay. Can we schedule that in by tomorrow?" she jokes.

"The slower you go, the faster you get there," I say, borrowing a phrase I once read. "We're talking about rewiring your brain."

Since that incident, Debra has continued to do better. She interacts with the staff. She takes direction. She converses with peers. Her progress is most apparent in her eyes, which are clear, present, and searching for connections. I can sense her aching for a chance to feel good.

"You know what else I miss?" she says.

"What?"

"My bed, my morning Starbucks, lunch at the Ivy . . . "

"Is that all? You mean sixteen days here isn't the Ritz Carlton?"

"I also miss my assistant. I wish he could've gone through all this for me. Then again, he's so tortured, he would've enjoyed it too much."

Through her malaise, Debra entertains me by poking fun at my favorite target, the media.

"This is where they should shoot a season of *Survivor*," she says. "I can see the two tribes. The stoners versus the tweakers." Translation: the pot addicts versus the amphetamine addicts.

"You're right," I laugh. "It has all the elements. Drugs. Drama. Fighting. Sex. Winners and losers."

"But do you think rehab is too five minutes ago?" she wonders. "Is my being here as passé as a Van Halen comeback?"

"I don't think you have to worry," I say. "As far as I'm concerned, the people who create the culture tend to be sick and have no idea what's real or healthy."

A vision bubbles through my head: the unmistakable voice of Robert Evans, the legendary Hollywood producer. Not long ago I listened to the audio edition of his celebrated autobiography, *The Kid Stays in the Picture,* and my reaction was a constant *Oh my God.* Evans was talented, to be sure. But a whole generation was influenced by him and his kind.

"I am surprised I haven't bumped into anyone I know," she says. "I thought all of Hollywood would be here."

"That's Malibu," I say.

Seeing her laugh reminds me why I am obsessed about my work, why I am on the radio five nights a week when I could be at home with my wife, why I speak at colleges, and why I'm so committed to making a difference in the quality of people's lives. I am not interested in telling people what to do. But I want to make them think about what's healthy and what's not, and perhaps encourage them to make better choices.

Sick people can feel better than they ever thought. Debra could be one of those people whom I'm able to draw back in from the abyss of pain and trouble. I can't predict her outcome. I guarantee she had no conscious idea that dealing with her drug habit would require a fearless confrontation with the trauma of past sexual abuse and other family problems. But she isn't flinching as she starts the journey.

"I have a question for you," she says.

"Shoot."

"When am I going to feel normal? When is all this crap inside me—this buzzing and dullness and pain and anxiety and the can't-sleep shit—going to stop?"

"It could take up to a year," I say.

Her eyes widen. "A whole fucking year?"

"And then you have the dysregulation of emotions from your past to deal with," I add.

"I should sue the fucking doctors who prescribed me those god-damn Vicodins and Somas in the first place."

"They thought they were helping you," I say. "Very few people understand this disease. From now on, it's going to be your responsibility."

About three hours later I walk out of a meeting with Dr. Finley, and he persuades me to take a brief stroll with him outside to take in the nice warm weather. Nothing is brief with Finley, though. He and his wife recently had their third child. This one, he says, is sleeping well, "so we're going to keep her."

He congratulates me on how much better contained Katherine is since I took away her cell phone, and then admits he switched his own cell phone to her plan.

We round a corner and I can't believe what I see ten yards in front of us.

Alexi is seated on a bench, smoking a cigarette.

We head right to her. I see her drop her hand with the cigarette behind her back, and when she brings it back up the cigarette is gone.

Her shame is so great she won't even acknowledge that we caught her smoking. This is truly funny.

"I can't believe you smoke!" I say.

"I don't," she replies.

"But we just saw you."

"I have two cigarettes a day. That's not smoking."

"What is it, then?" Finley asks.

"Relaxation."

"Could you relax in a different manner?" he asks, grinning.

Alexi sticks out her tongue and walks off.

That gets Finley and I talking about what motivates people to change their behavior. Finley reveals that he was once a two-pack-a-day smoker.

"You?" I say. "I'm shocked."

"Yeah. Then one day I just decided it was enough. I was going to stop."

"Like that? So abruptly?"

"Actually, I woke up one day and sent my wife out to get a pack of cigarettes. I was sick from not having them. While I waited for her to get back from the store, it occurred to me that this stuff had control over me, and *nothing* was going to have control over me."

"Then you stopped?"

"Yes."

"But wait. A lot of addicts realize things have control over them, and what do they do? They use more. As both of us know, even when addicts acknowledge something has control over them, they don't all of a sudden stop. It doesn't happen that way."

"I know," he says. "But I just decided nothing was going to control me."

We start walking back to the unit. For a moment or two I'm silent, thinking about what he's said.

"Wait a minute," I say. "You work with addicts all the time. You work with people who are controlled by drugs. People just don't decide to stop using drugs unless something really gets their attention. How were you able to make this massive change in your behavior?"

"I don't know," he says. "I just didn't want anything controlling me."

I'm confused and frustrated by his response. *He knows better,* I think to myself. There has to be something more, yet he's being so dismissive. I expect that kind of obfuscation from our patients, not from Finley.

We walk on in silence for a while. He doesn't seem to notice my frustration; he seems to be thinking about something. I'm reluctant to probe any further. Suddenly, as though thinking out loud, he begins telling me about his boyhood in Portugal. "When I was six years old my mother used to send me to the store by myself. I'd have to walk by the wharf, and the wharf was a hangout for alcoholics. As I'd go by, they'd reach out for me, yell things, threaten to throw me in a bag, and take me away."

"That sounds awful," I say.

"They scared the crap out of me," he continues. "We all heard stories about these drunks supposedly throwing sacks over kids, taking them away, and selling them into slavery. The poor kids would never see their parents again." He pauses a beat as if paralyzed by the memory of that fear. "These were scary guys, and alcohol seemed to make them that way. I came away from those experiences with an intense feeling that nothing would ever control me like that. So when I saw the cigarettes controlling me . . ."

"Not only that, but you aren't going to let it control anyone else. So now you have to cure all the alcoholics and addicts."

"Fascinating, isn't it?" he says. "I don't know what it is with human beings. Say a dog bites you when you're a child. Some people grow up avoiding dogs forever. But another side of the population becomes veterinarians."

"True," I say.

"Here's a thought, though. You didn't grow up in Portugal with drunks grabbing at you, and you're more into rescuing these patients than I am. Explain that?"

We are back at the unit. I put my hand on the door.

"Well?" he says. "No one has deeper need to rescue people than you. What's the story?"

"The man with the crosses in his eyes," I say.

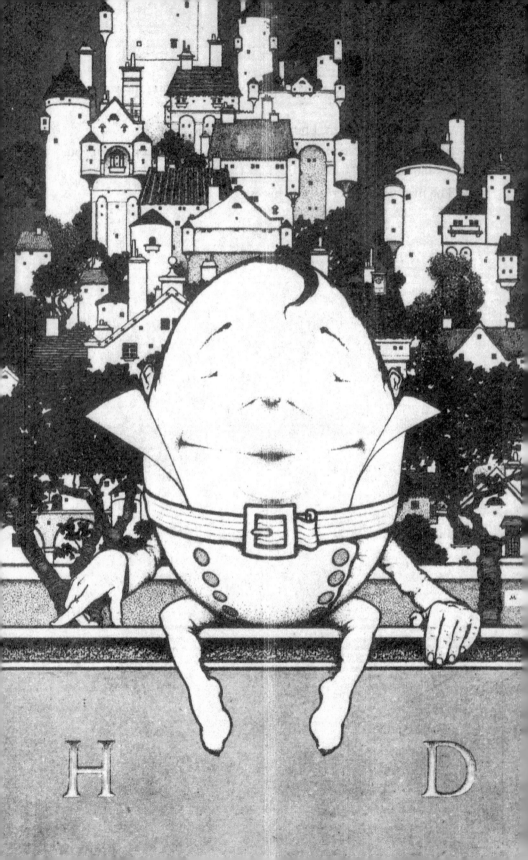

H
D

Three

AS A CHILD, I feared the man with the red crosses in his eyes. Until I was five years old, I had a recurring nightmare in which a man with red crosses in his eyes chased after my mother and me. We would be stuck in traffic, the two of us huddled in the passenger seat, while this guy came to get us, walking up and down cars behind us the way a tank would roll over them.

As an adult, I deciphered the dream. It turned out my mother had a miscarriage when I was only a year old. She had hemorrhaged severely, and was taken away in an ambulance—which in the late 1950s was a large white van with red crosses on the side. The man with the red crosses in his eyes bore a close resemblance to a neighbor who had taken care of me while my parents were at the hospital.

I was terrorized by the situation, and the helpless feeling I experienced lingered as a constant fear that bad things were about to happen to me.

Traumas like that leave imprints on parts of the brain that don't have a sense of time. The memory gives the sense that the trauma is always happening. As a result, I grew up with a feeling that there's a catastrophe waiting around every corner. I can't remember a time when I have not felt anxious. My response has been to try to control everything and everyone. I am a perfectionist. I rescue people. I have to make sure no one else gets carted away.

In reality, my childhood was pleasant and pain-free. The older of two children, I was raised in Pasadena by parents who valued stability and family. My father, Morton, was the son of a Chicago grocer who had escaped the pogroms in Russia, and then was nearly wiped out during the Great Depression. At eight, my dad got a job at a Chinese laundry to earn money for the family. As an adult, he became a doctor. He was a rescuer, too.

My mother, Helene, came from a highly Victorian upper-middle-class family in Philadelphia. She never saw her parents speak to each other. For instance, at the dinner table, her father would say to one of her sisters, "Please ask Mrs. Stansbury to pass the salt." She came to Hollywood in the early 1950s, and became a movie actress in film noir features until she married my father and had me.

She treated motherhood as a new career. My first year of life was defined by a symbiotic attachment to my mother. I was the sole object of her attention, and I reciprocated loyally with coos and smiles. As soon as I began walking, saying no, and having thoughts of my own, however, the narcissistic bubble burst, and I was cast out of Eden. Between the ages of two and three, I could swear, I remember a sense of terror, perhaps a remnant of the trauma of my mother's miscarriage. Eventually, though, we moved to a new house, and it was the good life. Things worked again.

But in those formative years, my brain was left with implicit wirings, structures that are literally like behavioral maps. In my case, I would grow up to be the perfect codependent, someone lured to the gratification of a fused relationship like the one I had with my mother at the start of my life.

As a teenager, I was a people pleaser. I had to be perfect for my parents out of fear of the old catastrophes that were subconsciously embedded in my brain. I couldn't do anything wrong out of fear it would devastate my parents. At Polytechnic High, I was a top student, captain of the football team, and the lead in the school play. For as long as I can remember, I assumed I would follow my dad into medicine, and so did everyone else.

The high school headmaster steered me toward science. In 1976 I enrolled at Amherst, a small private liberal arts college in Massachusetts. I majored in biology. By the end of the first term, I was miserable. As soon as the weather turned cold, I was second-guessing my decision to go to school in the East. Why was I freezing my ass off in New England when all I wanted was to be surfing and chasing girls at U.C. Santa Barbara? And how did I know I truly wanted to pursue medicine, anyway?

I brought my confusion home. During Christmas break, I announced at the dinner table that I no longer wanted to be a doctor. It was a good place for a scene. My parents nearly disowned me. Their anxiety overwhelmed me. This was the first time I had attempted to assert my independence, and it upset everything. It created catastrophe, just as I had feared. At the same time my high school girlfriend, to whom I'd clung desperately from 2,500 miles away, told me she wanted to see other guys. I was crushed; my world had fallen to pieces.

Back at school, I became depressed. The whole idea of the future was too much for me to handle, and I started having panic attacks. The first one came when I was rehearsing a play at Mount Holyoke College; I went back to my room convinced I was having a seizure. I thought I was going crazy. I struggled through the night, hoping I wasn't going to die, and in the morning I went to the student health center, where the psychologist appropriately recognized the signs of panic. He asked me to come back a few days later; I did. I was a lot better, but still anxious and complaining.

"I want you to see a doctor," he said.

I saw a doctor. He checked me out and told me to take a walk. He didn't know squat about depression, and he missed the whole thing.

For the next year and a half, I struggled without support, searching myself as best I could, and during that time I decided for myself to pursue science. The lack of structure in my life bothered me; so did the lack of purpose. I realized I needed both. I didn't know it, but that's where my need to make a difference began. I threw myself into my books, and responded to the challenges of an outstanding group of professors. I rededicated myself to becoming a doctor. This time, though, the decision was all mine.

In 1980 I entered medical school at USC, where my zeal as an overachiever paid off. For two years, I worked my ass off. The real learning began in year three, with practical experience. During my first rotation in the Neurological ICU, for instance, the resident led me and several other students into the unit early in the morning and issued a complex list of instructions. "This patient needs a Swan. That one an A-line. The next patient gets a ventriculostomy..." Then he departed, explaining, "I'll be in surgery all day. See you at seven."

I had no idea what he was talking about. None of us did. But we opened packages. We read the instruction manuals. We figured it out.

Other lessons were harder to figure out. One day, while I was working in the general hospital ward at County General, the city's dumping ground for the sick and destitute, I saw a black woman in her twenties who'd been shot through her abdomen. Sitting up in bed, she was suffering through a terrible, unimaginable pain in total silence, writhing, waiting for someone to help her. I had stopped by her bed, hoping to alleviate her pain, when the supervising surgical resident said, "Leave her. We've got cases that are more urgent than hers."

I put down her chart. He was right. A bullet through the abdomen wasn't the worst case. It was nothing. Something that would wait till morning. There were people who were worse, people who had been run over by cars or stabbed in gang fights, people with multiple gun-shot wounds, people who wouldn't survive if they didn't get immediate attention. And this was the judgment residents had to develop in a MASH unit like this.

As we walked away, he said, "You'll get used to it. You'll learn to do it."

I thought, *No, I won't.*

I was wrong. I very quickly saw more than I ever imagined, and came to realize that doctors are basically biological repairmen, especially in inner-city hospitals on violence-riddled Saturday nights. On my first night at County General, I treated a guy with a penis the size of a foot-ball. It turned out he'd been shot in the ass, and the bullet had exited through his penis. After a few Saturdays, though, I learned that two things could be predicted with 100 percent accuracy: If you asked any-one with a knife wound what happened, they'd say, "I don't know." And if a person had something stuck up their butt—which in my expe-rience included lightbulbs, broomsticks, and grapefruits—they'd explain, "It was an accident. I sat on it."

For a while, I was headed toward a specialty in orthopedics. If you had an athletic background, which I did, the ortho team drafted you. I liked the physicality of it. As it turned out, though, ortho was where I treated my first addicts and alcoholics. They are generally thrill-seekers who like motorcycles and fast cars and extreme sports. They also like to experience these things while they're loaded. They get into accidents. I remember in particular one biker whose leg had been man-gled below his knee in a crash. He had a pin through his tibia, and he was in traction—his leg was up on a pulley. But what you saw was a bone with a foot on the end, and his calf muscle hanging down from the leg. Every day we chipped a bit of dead bone off his leg. The whole spectacle was revolting.

I saw on his chart that he was a heroin addict. One day I told him he should quit.

"You're right," he said sincerely. "But I'm in excruciating pain. Can I get some more morphine?"

He genuinely needed it. He was a mess. "Let me see what I can do," I said.

I got him more, and seeing it do its job was equally satisfying for me. Early in your training as a doctor, you don't have a lot of skills. One thing you can do is take away pain with opiates. I was very gratified.

In the early 1980s, there wasn't much knowledge about treating addicts, and though my training routinely exposed me to hundreds of junkies, dopers, meth freaks, pill-poppers, and alcoholics, I would end up advising addicts that what they needed was a new set of friends. I told dozens of alcoholics to just stop drinking.

The residents and the attendings threw up their hands; they just got frustrated with the addicts, and after a while they gave up even telling them they should stop. They wouldn't even address it. I hated being ineffectual. I saw young alcoholics returning again and again after we had told them they would die if they didn't quit. They didn't care about stopping. They wanted more meds. Why didn't they listen to what we said?

Then I started moonlighting at Las Encinas. Though it was located in the heart of old Pasadena, somehow I had never heard of it. But I came to know it very quickly. As a young internist, I performed all the basic medical care for the psychiatric patients, and soon I discovered that the patients with the most medical needs were the addicts.

Las Encinas was unique among hospitals. It had a detox protocol and program for treatment of the addict. Dr. Mike Meyers, a trailblazer in addiction medicine, had established one of California's first comprehensive chemical dependency units at the hospital. Meyers was able to withdraw addicts systematically. He had turned detox into a clinical discipline. Up to this time, detoxing patients had been very haphazard and often just plain dangerous.

The more I observed, the more I wanted to know. Steadily and naturally, I gravitated toward the chemical dependency unit. After a year and half of moonlighting, I began to feel adept at helping patients through withdrawal. In the beginning, though, it was difficult. I dubbed myself (none too proudly, I might add) Dr. Pushover for how easily I was manipulated by addicts, who I soon realized are the smartest and shrewdest patients in a hospital when it comes to getting what they want. No patients were better at it than Anna and Elena Petrovic, sisters and longtime opiate addicts from Greece. They were in their mid-twenties. Anna was an opiate addict, and Elena was a speed addict. They loved me. I was their favorite doctor. Every time they had an ache or pain, anxiety, or trouble sleeping, they could count on me to help them out. "Don't worry," I said. "I'll get you something."

Elena came and left without ever having a breakthrough. Anna struggled. She kept relapsing but coming back. Finally, on her third time, she declared herself done with drugs. By this time I knew her pretty well and saw that something about her was different. It was all in her eyes. They struck me as depleted, frightened, and from what I could discern, either she was truly done, or she'd soon be dead.

I asked what happened.

Sobbing uncontrollably, Anna described how less than twenty-four hours earlier she had been scoring heroin at her dealer's house when a gunfight had broken out. The dealer had given her a gun and told her to shoot anyone who came into the room. Instead, Anna had rolled beneath a bed and put the gun in her mouth. Scared, crying, and desperately intent on removing herself from this nightmare, she had tried summoning the nerve to pull the trigger, but she couldn't do it.

That was the end of the line, the point at which she had two choices: death or recovery. She saw it and felt it. That was her bottom.

"I took it as far as I could," she later told me. "If I don't want to die, I have to get better."

About ten years later, I bumped into Anna at the store. She had two kids, drove a minivan, and had married an engineer. Her sister was still out.

I couldn't help but ask what the difference was that allowed her to change and not her sister.

"I just got it," she said, and then shrugged. "I don't know how else to explain it."

Neither do I.

One of the toughest lessons I learned in those early days came from the person who taught me more about addicts than almost anyone. Betty was one of the unit's star counselors, a former heroin addict who'd been through treatment numerous times, including several stints before Dr. Meyers created the chemical dependency unit, and she had a magical touch when it came to working with other addicts. Not only did she know all the tricks, she had a sixth sense that I envied.

"Count your blessings," she said one day when I wished I knew what she did. "You got your knowledge from medical school, not from shooting up in bathrooms like me."

Then she told me a story from the days when she was trying to get sober before she got in the program. Like all heroin addicts, she was convinced all she had to do to get well was to get off the heroin. She hatched a plan to "explore her roots" in Czechoslovakia. She was convinced that would keep her sober. (In drug treatment circles, this is what's known as "a geographic"—moving away from the physical scene of your drug use.)

It never works. On her way to Prague, Betty had a short stopover in London. She decided to spend the downtime at the National Gallery, taking in an exhibition. As Betty told me, she felt terrific on the flight over. She was on her way to the promised land. She wasn't even thinking about drugs. Yet within an hour of getting to the museum she was slamming heroin in a bathroom with a security guard she spotted in the main gallery. She didn't even introduce herself. She just went up to him and said, "Let's go."

"How'd you know to seek out the guard?" I asked. "You were in a room in a museum—why would you walk up to a guy with a gun? In a uniform?" I was mystified.

"If you're an addict," she said, "you just know. The drive to use is so powerful, you develop an extrasensory ability."

After that relapse, she got into the program, listened to direction, and became a star in the treatment field. Still, though she was a counselor for years, her disease eventually came back for her. The first sign was trouble at work. After years of dependable, consistent, and conscientious work, she changed. She started splitting people, pitting one against the other. She complained about her superiors. She became erratic. She may not have been using then; it might just have been time for her to get a new job. It was clear that she was no longer happy; she needed a change. But the whole process of leaving resurrected feelings of abandonment and loss that overwhelmed her.

I, of course, defended her, made excuses for her, ever the good codependent. I could see her emotional chaos emerging, but I thought it was just the difficulty she was having leaving a place and a team to which she'd felt so connected. She had worked with us all ever since she got sober; I knew it was painful for her to contemplate moving on.

One day Betty called me as I sat completing some paperwork in my office. She sounded breathless and desperate. "I need to see you right away."

Alarmed by the distress in her voice, I told her to come right over. She flew into my office, closed the door, and dropped into a chair. I had become used to her complaining to me about how others were to blame for how she was feeling. I figured she was going to go off about one of the nurses who was nearby. But today she seemed different. I was immediately anxious.

Then she leaned forward, in a manner that made me uncomfortable and blurted out, "I need to have you—right now."

Almost reflexively I shot back, "That is just not possible." And, strangely, I felt a flood of guilt and confusion.

"You see," she said. "I know that about you. That's what makes you so great. That's what makes me want you."

I just sat there shaking my head, feeling incredibly uncomfortable, not knowing what else to do but apologize. At that point in my career it was difficult for me to set limits. I felt guilty and apologetic for exposing her to shame. I was uncomfortable not being able to comply with someone else's needs, even when they were completely out of line. And yet, of course, I could do nothing to answer them.

A few pleasantries followed. She tried to joke away the discomfort. She was clearly somewhat ashamed, but like most addicts, she wouldn't stay with that feeling long. She slipped out as quickly as she blew in.

In retrospect, I didn't think it all the way through. I followed my own human reaction, rather than recognizing an addict's behavior for what it was.

Two months later, still in the throes of her bad behavior, she approached me in the parking lot and showed me a picture of her naked ass with welts all over it.

"You should check this out," she said. "A riding crop. That will really pin your pupils."

Such behavior was so far out of character for the Betty I knew—the consummate professional she had been for years. Today, such conduct would never get past me. I know too much about this disease and its cunning ways. At that point, though, I was still mystified. I tried talking to her, but she wouldn't open the door to any honest communication. Within six months, she left and found a job at a different facility, where she got involved with a man early in his recovery. (Another common pattern: People with long-term sobriety who relapse usually do so after a bad relationship choice.) A few months after she took her new job, I got a call from her father. Betty was dead; according to him, she had shot herself in the chest with her boyfriend's gun.

I must admit that I've never quite been able to accept that story; the Betty I knew was never suicidal, never self-destructive. Even today, it seems more likely to me that someone turned a gun on her. The boyfriend also ended up in the hospital with self-inflicted gunshot wounds. What are we supposed to believe—that it was a double suicide? Whether it was a case of foul play or not, however, this much is true: Ultimately the disease was the true cause of death.

Betty was the first addict I had become close to and then lost, and the news shook me in a profound way. My job was to save people, to prevent catastrophe, and here one had occurred to someone close to me. But it was too painful for me to accept the full force of the situation. And so I carried on, returning to my role at Las Encinas, still trying to pull people away from death and toward a place where they might start to felt better again. Even in the face of evidence that I might not be good enough, I still had to believe I could prevent bad things from happening.

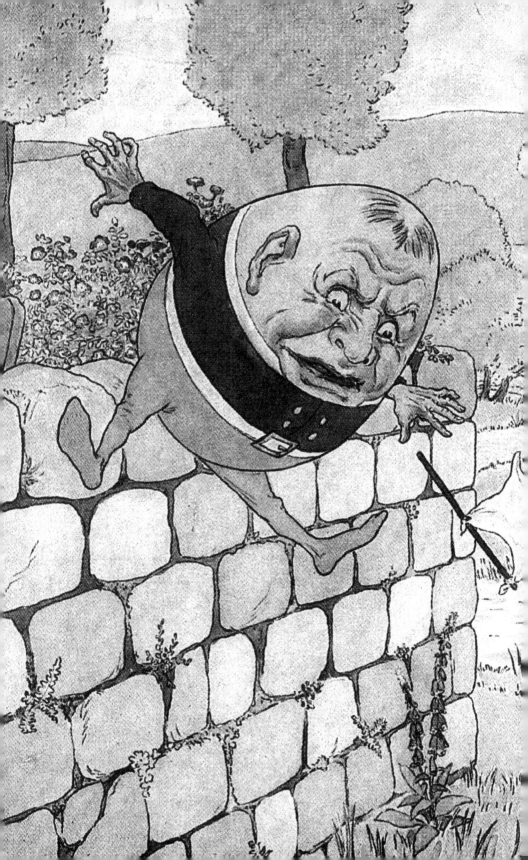

Four

IT'S AFTERNOON, AND I'm in the conference room with a TV crew, tap-ing a discussion I'm having with "Science Guy" Bill Nye about ad-diction. There's a loud commotion somewhere outside the hospital entrance, and we wait a long time for things to calm down. It sounds like a patient problem, though, so I excuse myself to go out and lend a hand.

Several people from the front-end admitting staff are out there, try-ing to calm down a woman I immediately recognize as a former patient named Rebecca. She is very thin, blond, and flushed with anger. She's clearly on something, and she's screaming about being ripped off by the hospital.

"I want my money," she says.

I see several patients glance out their windows.

"What money?" I ask, closing the distance between us.

"The money I left in the hospital safe."

Rebecca's the poster girl for the notion that bad things happen to good people. At twenty-eight, she's attractive and smart as hell. She began to drink heavily while studying to be a dietician. After a year or two working in a hospital, she was struggling to keep it together. She soon went from alcohol to coke, and then into rehab at least twice. Though Rebecca would do the first of AA's twelve steps, admitting she was powerless and that her life had become unmanageable, she wouldn't capitulate to the process, and then she would come back for treatment.

Most recently she had spent a month at the unit, then six weeks at Sober Living, a halfway home where the structure from rehab is continued and reinforced in a less intensive setting. While in Sober Living, she continued to attend our day programs. She had followed instructions so well there that I thought she'd finally gotten it. In the midst of recovery, though, she was diagnosed with breast cancer. The blow sent her reeling back to the bottle, and then to the hospital.

I was crushed to see her back in the unit. Not by the fact that she'd relapsed: Her addiction was something we could deal with. The fear that had gripped her—that was something else.

Rebecca detoxed quickly, returned to Sober Living, and seemed buoyed by my repeated assurances that women her age with breast cancer did very well with the most aggressive treatment possible. The odds were in her favor. That was three weeks earlier.

Now Rebecca and I are standing in the sun on a warm afternoon. She appears to have lost at least twenty pounds since I last saw her. Her skin is chafed and sunburned. She's filthy.

"Hey, it's me here," I say. "We can talk."

I have trouble getting her to track and stay with me, but she calms down.

I try a different approach. "How's the cancer treatment going?" I say, knowing this is the heart of her relapse.

She looks up at me. Right in my eyes.

"Two of my lymph nodes tested positive," she says.

"Which we'd discussed as a possibility. And so?"

"My doctors recommended the most aggressive treatment, chemo and radiation."

"Again, we already knew this."

She adds a new wrinkle. Someday she wants to have children, and she's worried that the radiation and tamoxifen will make her infertile. Should she harvest her eggs, she asks, and save them? Or not? Should she just have the treatment?

These are good questions, and heavy issues for anyone. Still, I don't sense that we've touched on the real issue, the one that set her off.

"What happened right before you started using again?" I ask.

I'm quiet, willing to wait. I try never to let myself get in the way of my patients.

"I was getting an MRI, at least I was supposed to, but they couldn't get the IV hooked up," says Rebecca. What followed was a gut-wrenching debacle: When the X-ray techs were unable to find a vein, they cancelled her MRI and delayed her cancer treatment, which freaked her out and caused her to start drinking again. With that first drink she picked up where her disease had left off and got worse, ending up on the street.

"I can feel the cancer in me," she says, breaking down into tears. "I—I don't want to die. I'm scared."

"I understand," I say, taking some tissues off the counter and handing them to her. "It's a scary thing. But you aren't dying. You're trying to get treatment. Let's focus on that. You have to get through this."

Rebecca loses focus and grows agitated again. "I can't. I mean, I don't know how anymore."

I feel her frustration, fear, and the abyss of powerlessness, the deep, dark dungeon of pain that is at the core of so many addicts' use.

"You can. And for starters, you have to get back to Sober Living."

"I don't have any money," she cries.

Suddenly Rebecca turns away and heads for the parking lot. She drives a black VW Jetta with a dent on the passenger door. The driver's seat is occupied by a friend of hers, who tells me that he's risking a lot to help Rebecca. He looks very frightened and overwhelmed. He's a former coke addict on probation, he says; he could go back to jail for being around a person using drugs or alcohol.

"But I didn't want to leave her," he says. "She's in a really bad place."

"Yeah," I agree.

I didn't anticipate someone else in the picture, but he could be an asset. At this point, the situation could go either way. As I explain to them, Rebecca could continue losing control until her deepest fears turn prophetic, or else she can get help. She needs to get back to Sober Living, where she had been doing well.

"Rebecca, will you go if your friend takes you there?" I ask.

She shrugs her shoulders and looks at the ground.

I can't imagine what's going on in her head. Her thoughts are so jumbled. This kind of resistance is something I have trouble coming to terms with.

She doesn't know where to turn. She needs someone else to provide the structure.

I look at her friend. "Will you take her there now, and promise me that you'll see her get checked in and situated?"

He nods.

I open the passenger door and help Rebecca into the car.

"This is going to be okay," I say. "You're going to be fine."

Then they drive off.

A few hours later Rebecca is back, defeated and desperate. She had been readmitted to the hospital after being turned away from Sober Living. When I ask why, she says they wanted her to detox before they let her back in. She stands in silence outside the nursing station, helpless, crying, waiting for me to tell her what to do. I don't always know what that should be. But then something happens.

Alexi turns the corner and talks to Rebecca.

"Just put her in a bed and we'll let her detox," says Alexi. "Then we'll send her back to Sober Living."

"But I don't have any money," says Rebecca.

"I'll figure something out," I say.

"Thank you," she says.

Rebecca stays for the next three days. By then her brain starts working again, and she is able to return to Sober Living. She requires hardly any withdrawal medication. Simply being in the hospital's safe environment enables her to reconstitute. She can't remember the scene she had outside the hospital. Before she leaves, we have a nice talk and agree that cancer sucks.

"But you deal with it head-on and, given the facts, you have a good chance of going into remission."

"I really have to get my shit together this time." She chuckles. "I would say the same thing to my patients at work. 'You have to get your shit together and decrease the animal fats and sodium.' "

"Then you know how hard it is," I say. "You also know it can be done."

"Yeah. Sometimes."

At 6:30 P.M., I'm standing in front of a blackboard, watching a lecture hall fill up. About seventy-five patients, former patients, and their families, partners, and friends—some with several days of sobriety, others with many years—are seated in rows of metal folding chairs in a small bungalow a short stroll from the unit. They represent all types, from businessmen to bikers, homemakers to high school students. They have come to listen to my weekly medical lecture, an in-depth discussion about their disease and its effect on their biology.

The hourlong presentation is aimed at giving them more insight into their disease. Few of them really understand addiction. They don't know the roots of its biology. They don't know why addiction is a disease. If asked why they use, they offer some variation of "I'm fucked up." If asked why they can't stop using, they reply, "I'm fucked up." They cannot see themselves as anything but victims. I believe information is power. The more people understand, the less inclined they will be to blame themselves.

I start by asking, "Who can tell me the difference between abuse and addiction?" That begins a lively discussion. Eventually we conclude that abuse is "the use of any potentially harmful substance with no therapeutic value that affects the brain," and addiction is "the continued use of a substance in spite of consequences." They should give themselves a pat on the back, I tell them: It took the world's brightest scientists decades to figure that one out. We did it in a few minutes.

"Now let me ask a harder question," I say. "Can anyone define *disease?* Before you can say you suffer from a disease, you should know what one is."

This sparks another lively discussion. Though it reveals how little average people know about biology, it is also a tough question. Until recently, experts didn't understand much more than the layman about the secret relationship between drugs, the brain, biology, and disease. Think about it: For decades, drug abusers and alcoholics were thought of as people with low self-control. Even scientists and doctors thought they could control their problems by exercising more willpower. How many addicts were told to change their friends, move neighborhoods, or take a different way home so they wouldn't pass the liquor store?

It got worse. For years, addicts were thought to be morally deficient people who could be saved if they would simply acknowledge and change their sinful ways. Well, in reality, no matter what they acknowledge, addicts can't just stop. That is addiction—the inability to stop, no matter what. Addicts know every consequence of their addiction: lost jobs, screwed-up relationships, squandered money, betrayed relatives, and so on. But they can't help their behavior.

Eventually, though, studies began to show that addicts suffered from a disease, rather than a lack of self-control. And clinicians working with addicts and alcoholics began to recognize the difficulty addicts had in quitting. After former First Lady Betty Ford went public with her drinking problem in the late 1970s, there was wider familiarity, understanding, and even sympathy for people who checked into the Betty Ford Center, Hazelden, Cedar Hills, and other rehab facilities seeking treatment for alcoholism and drug addiction.

But misperceptions lingered. With the growth in the number of treatment facilities, many came to believe these problems could be cleared up in a mere twenty-eight days. But further study has shown the disease to be much more complex. By the early 1990s, new research allowed addiction to be defined more specifically as a biological disorder with a genetic basis, plus progressive use in the face of adverse consequences, and denial of a problem. More recent findings have focused on the relationship between addiction and the drives in the deepest brain structures that are outside of conscious volitional control.

As I talk about this, though, I can see some eyes in the audience start to glaze over. All that scientific jargon—this is starting to sound like school. So I change tack.

"I'm really talking about three things," I say. "Why you use drugs. Why you get addicted. And how you get better. Let's start with why you use. Any guesses?"

"It feels good," a young Latino teenager in front says.

"It lets me escape," an alcoholic woman with a few years' sobriety says from the middle of the room.

"Because if I'd done what I really wanted to do, I'd be in jail for killing my father," a middle-aged man adds. He gets a knowing laugh.

I allow that all those answers are correct. "A healthy person, whether he realizes it or not, populates his emotional world with soothing or reassuring images that can be called upon in times of distress, need, or aloneness. But the individual who has suffered trauma during his formative years retreats from the world as a result of that abuse." I pause. "Look around the room. Think of the people in treatment with you and those in your AA groups. What do you all have in common?"

"Bic lighters," someone jokes.

"Fucked-up lives," someone else says.

"Be more specific," I say.

"Fucked-up parents," a college-age girl calls out.

"We're just fucked up," a guy says.

"You want to know the common denominator among my patients?" I say, turning serious. "They all had traumatic experiences in early life that caused them to feel helpless, powerless, and in grave danger." I see some people nodding. "This feeling of helplessness creates an inability to process feelings and an aversion to exploring other minds. There's no trust. If you can't trust, you can't connect with anyone. Without the capacity to activate the part of the brain that allows for connection and exploration of other people, an individual loses the main mechanism for discovering who we are and the ability to regulate emotions.

"Think about it," I continue. "For all of us, other people function as self-regulating agents. We learn to identify ourselves when we recognize ourselves in others. We constantly think, 'Oh, that's exactly how I feel.' Or you say, 'I was thinking that exact same thing.' Our experiences of ourselves become internalized as a result of this sort of interaction. We figure out who we are.

"But my patients—many of you—automatically take the emotional posture that the abuse you fell victim to was your fault. Why? Because at least then you avoid feeling the threat of the contents of the mind of your abuser. You don't ask why Daddy hits you or Mommy's passed out on the living room floor. If it's your fault, you're more in control.

"You're sacrificing yourself in order to maintain the illusion of control in a situation that otherwise you'd experience as irrational and unpredictable. Of course, if you're at fault, you're also feeling shame. In addition, your brain kicks into an automatic biological response that becomes a permanent mechanism for dealing with interpersonal stress.

This is the action your brain takes to escape these situations from which there's no escape, something called dissociation."

A gray-haired man in mechanic's coveralls raises his hand. I have treated him and his son.

"So what are you saying that I'm feeling?" he asks.

"What did I say all my patients have in common?"

"Helplessness," he says.

"What do you feel when you're helpless?" I ask.

"Fear," he says.

"Right. The initial response to threat is fear. How does this happen? Well, chemicals flood into the brain as the flight-or-fight response is initiated. When escape seems hopeless, your brain switches into shut-down mode, releasing a flood of endorphins that provide a soothing numbness as you wait for the inevitable to occur.

"The experience that predominates this reaction is what?"

I call on a young guy seated on the side.

"I don't even get what you're saying," he says. "But I'm guessing that it's the sense that you're somewhere else, gone, shut down."

"Exactly," I say. "Dissociation. You separate and isolate yourself from the world, from feelings, from others. While such a reaction may protect you from the horrifying experience—whatever that turns out to be—the price is a long-term difficulty in integrating emotional experiences. Think back to whatever age you suffered trauma. That's when you shut down. That's when you decided you were to blame. That's when you stopped developing and growing in the part of the brain that regulates emotions. That's when you stopped connecting with others."

"You know what picture I'm getting?" a man in front says. "I see one of those Japanese soldiers coming out of the jungle after hiding for thirty years because he didn't know the war had ended. You don't know anything that's going on. You don't know who to trust or which side you're on. Your instinct would be to turn around and run back into the jungle, where it was safe."

"Kind of," I say. "But let me go on. So what happens? The personality that accompanies you as you mature physically tends to have a hard time in relationships. In fact, the original victimization is often recreated over and over again. It's the same problem repeated, and more problems ensue. You can't trust someone with your tender needs in a genuine relationship. Why? It's too dangerous. It's too likely to expose you to trauma again.

"So your ability to develop brain mechanisms to regulate emotions is impaired, since we tend to build these through intimate connections with others. It's a great big mess that causes you to enter your young life looking for solutions to those feelings of being, as most of you say, fucked up. You aren't able to find any peace until you find drugs or alcohol. Then, suddenly, for the first time, everything seems all right."

I see heads nod.

"Are you with me still?"

I get a chorus of yesses.

"Good. We just talked about the consequences of trauma, which basically set the stage for the addictive process. Let's go to the next point: Why are you addicted? The simple answer is that some people are configured biologically in such a way to respond very positively to substances. That's what gets you using. But what makes you an addict is primarily a change in a tiny region of the brain called the nucleus accumbens.

"This region of your brain has started to mistake the chemical message of survival with the message delivered by drugs. The drive to use becomes confused with the drive to survive. This drive overwhelms the centers of the brain where cognitive reasoning and will reside. This shouldn't be confused with the feel-good part of addiction. These are powerful drives that begin emanating from deep nonverbal drive centers of the brain and demand gratification with the same life-or-death intensity as taking a breath. This is what keeps you using even when it doesn't feel good or work for you anymore.

"Interestingly, a certain percentage of people feel shitty when they're exposed to endorphinlike substances."

"Then they aren't real addicts," a black woman who's been in and out of treatment several times says.

"That's partly true," I say. "I had a patient come in with uncontrollable sobbing from, of all drugs, Vicodin."

"Oh, please," she says, waving me off.

"You're like my addict patients," I say.

"No, I *am* one of your addict patients," she laughs.

"My addict patients feel incredible when they're exposed to opiates or any other chemical that tickles the brain's endogenous morphine system, like alcohol, cocaine, sometimes pot—"

"Heroin," someone chimes.

"Yes. In fact, all drugs of addiction have in common that they stimulate the endorphin system. That's the feel-good part of drugs. So these people configured to respond positively to substance feel great when they're using. So great they keep using to regulate their emotional lives. As time goes by, all drugs of addiction cause depletion of brain chemicals."

"What?" one of my more vocal participants asks.

"The endorphin system alters itself in response to months or years of saturation, and so when the drugs are removed the brain is no longer able to screen out discomfort or pain. This of course happens at a time when the patient is trying to come to terms with the pain of acknowledging the consequences of the disease—destroyed relationships, legal problems, health issues, and so on. Not only is the endorphin system altered; the mood center, serotonin, is also depleted, as is the anxiety-regulating GABA system and the stress chemical cortisol. All are profoundly abnormal from drug use, leaving the patient in an impaired and terribly unpleasant brain state."

"Welcome to my world," a guy yells out.

He gets a big laugh.

"Remember, you've relied on drugs to deal with unpleasant or over-whelming emotions often since adolescence. Those same emotional conditions that started you using have remain unchanged. Not only that, the drugs have blocked you from tackling the usual milestones of development. There's even some evidence that certain of these drugs actually impair the brain's growth. And, finally, many of these drugs of addiction damage the brain, leaving biological impairments that affect mood, anxiety regulation, and memory.

"So you enter sobriety with this incredible set of biological and often psychological and developmental circumstances stacked against you. Throw in the misery of withdrawal, the social shame and stigma associated with the disease, the consequences of your behavior, and on top of everything the fact that you really love to do drugs—well, it's no wonder people relapse."

"Amen," the black woman says, to a mix of laughs and clapping.

"But here's the fascinating—or depressing—part," I continue. "This is not the disease itself. What I've described are merely factors that come to bear on the disease. The disease is a disorder of the drive centers of the brain—specifically the so-called mesolimbic reward center, as I've explained, in the nucleus accumbens. That part of the brain is deep in the reptilian core. It doesn't have language or logic. Just as with lower life forms, it exists merely to increase the drive that activates behavior fostering survival. It's the survival center, and it's gone awry.

"I'll give you an example. Every cocaine addict knows that he or she will never get the same high they got from their first hit off the pipe. In fact, they feel shittier and shittier with each hit, yet they continue to use until they're floridly psychotic, sitting in a dark room by them-selves, peeking out through the curtains at the black helicopters they imagine are hovering overhead."

"It was army men for me," a guy in a blue suit says.

"I heard paramilitary spacemen hiding in the bushes," a car me-chanic seated nearby adds.

"The point is, you continue to use because the drive centers command you to use. Your brain's rational understanding is overwhelmed. Though you know perfectly well that you won't get high and will end up feeling like shit, you can't stop. You can't stop, no matter how hard you try or how badly you want to. That's addiction.

"There's a lot of new science being done in this area, but basically what we have here is a set of very powerful drives being activated beneath conscious control in a region of the brain that can't be influenced by reason, language, or will. We have a terrible time in this country accepting disorders of will. How often do you hear someone explain their behavior by saying, 'Hey, it's a free country.' But as you well know, you're not free from the grips of the biology of this region of the brain and the effect the disease has on it."

I know this is all still pretty technical material, but I can feel a sense of excitement in the room, a tangible buzz as those listening acquire new or additional understanding about why they really are powerless over their addiction. Why does that create such a reaction? Because the first of the twelve steps in Alcoholics Anonymous is admitting that you are powerless over your disease. Now they can really believe it's true, and we can start discussing how you get better.

"Powerlessness," I say, gazing across the room to emphasize that each one of them has this in common. "What kind of feeling does that evoke in you?"

"Pain," a young man in the back of the room says without hesitation.

I nod, smiling. I know the young man well: Patrick, a patient of mine who's recently turned twenty. He's been doing well in recovery. He's even returned to college.

"I just feel pain," he continued.

"Can I use you as an example?" I ask, aware that he has shared in previous groups with many in the room. He says yes, and I encourage him to fill us in on the details. Raised the only child of an alcoholic father and addicted mother, Patrick was on his own from the time he could walk. His life had little structure. He was neglected by his parents and abused by neighbors. He started smoking pot at the age of ten.

Two years later he was on to coke. He was thirteen when his father died. His mother floated in and out, either ignorant of or indifferent to his drug use. By sixteen he was using speed. Still, against seemingly insurmountable odds, he managed to get into a city college. He was a major control freak—anything to avoid the instability of his childhood—and yet he couldn't control his drug use.

"It was like I was running all the time," he says. "Even when I was asleep I was still running."

"Running from what?" I ask.

"The pain."

"A specific pain?"

"No, not really. It's more like a feeling of pain that blankets everything. It's just always there. My whole deal has been avoidance through control."

He had articulated something that's key: the fact that the pain that started with the traumas of his childhood was still ongoing in the present. It still felt raw and fresh. It had happened then, it was happening now, and as far as his brain was concerned it was going to keep happening into the future. He was in what some call the "running" phase of post-traumatic stress disorder.

They have no idea how much I relate personally. But ever since I saw the man with the red crosses in his eyes following my mother's miscarriage, I've felt—no, I've known—that bad things are happening to me. Period. Then, now, and always. Like Patrick, I've tamed those feelings by maintaining control, striving for perfection, rescuing people. I even have a job where bad shit happens every day. It's exhausting.

If I'd had the genetic disposition, I would've made a great addict.

"You can see how as a result of those early traumas you have difficulty trusting and opening up to another person," I say. "If you're a kid, why would you trust ever again? But without that capacity to trust, you can't get an accurate read on your own self. You never learn how to regulate your own feelings."

A hand rises from the middle, and a husky man with bushy sideburns and tattooed arms stands up to speak. "How do you learn?" he asks.

"That's the getting-it part of recovery. You have to be willing—willing to follow directions, willing to trust, willing to form connections, willing to explore feelings. That's the essence of recovery, of the twelve steps," I say. "In recovery, you learn how to regulate your emotions without getting high. This is where you learn connection, the connection you didn't learn when it was interrupted by trauma in childhood. The real work gets done when you sit down with a sponsor and trust that that person will be available without shaming or intruding as you express genuine and tender needs. Then, instead of suffering rejection, you experience relief and gradually a new sense of self. It's only through relationships with others that we develop a sense of who we are and the ability to regulate our emotions."

Afterward, as people drift outside to smoke and chat among themselves, I am taken almost by force into a corner by one of my regulars, Rosie, a thirty-two-year-old blonde from Cheviot Hills, a suburb of shopping malls and carpools south of Beverly Hills. I'd spotted her during the lecture, sitting in the second-to-the-last row, rocking so furiously it's a miracle she didn't fly off her chair. Eight months sober after treatment for a Klonopin addiction, she's still having a rough time, which isn't unusual—though by staying clean this long she's already surpassed some expectations around the unit.

Rosie is an unlikely-looking addict. The mother of two, married to a lawyer, she goes to the gym, does yoga, drives a BMW X5. After she was brought into the unit, we even discovered that we knew people in common through our children's sports activities. At one point during her hospitalization she turned to me, crying, "I don't get how this could happen to me," she said. "I'm a healthy person."

Healthy, except that her parents were alcoholics, her childhood chaotic. In order to survive, she had to sacrifice her own emotional development by caring for her raging parents. As an adult, she was hyperbusy with her family and career. Eventually she began having panic attacks. A doctor put her on Klonopin to regulate her anxiety, and over time she started gobbling the downers by the fistful, until they overtook her life.

This conscientious wife and mother of two was brought into the hospital by concerned neighbors. She stayed four weeks, the first two of which were spent going through the absolutely hellish withdrawal that's typical of Klonopin addicts: severe pain, constant panic, extreme agitation.

She continues to wrestle with the symptoms of low-level withdrawal, which can linger for a year or more. As she's told me in the past, she can't believe she isn't feeling better yet.

And now?

I set up two chairs for us in the corner and sit down.

"It's really bad," she says. "I'm always speedy. I break out into sweats. It won't let go of me, and I need some relief."

"Tell me how bad it is right now on a scale of one to ten."

"Four."

"What was it yesterday?"

"Three."

I put my hand on her shoulder.

"Maybe next week you'll be down to a two."

"But sometimes I feel like I'm literally going to go out of my mind."

"That's to be expected. You're going to have to deal with that for a while as your brain's chemistry settles down and returns to normal. It takes a very long time."

She sighs.

"But look, you're doing what's necessary, you're hanging tough, and that's a good thing."

"But I'm going crazy."

"I'd argue the opposite. To me, mental health isn't always about feeling good. Nor is it always about avoiding depression. Nor about being happy. As I define it, mental health is about accepting reality on reality's terms. And I think you're doing just that."

"Yeah, but it's a day-by-day proposition."

"That's the idea."

Then we're both silent. There's nothing left to say. Rosie looks straight at me, a direct, healthy look that communicates everything I want to see from someone in recovery—strength, determination, connection. I give her hand a gentle squeeze of support. Then we're done, at least I hope, until the following week.

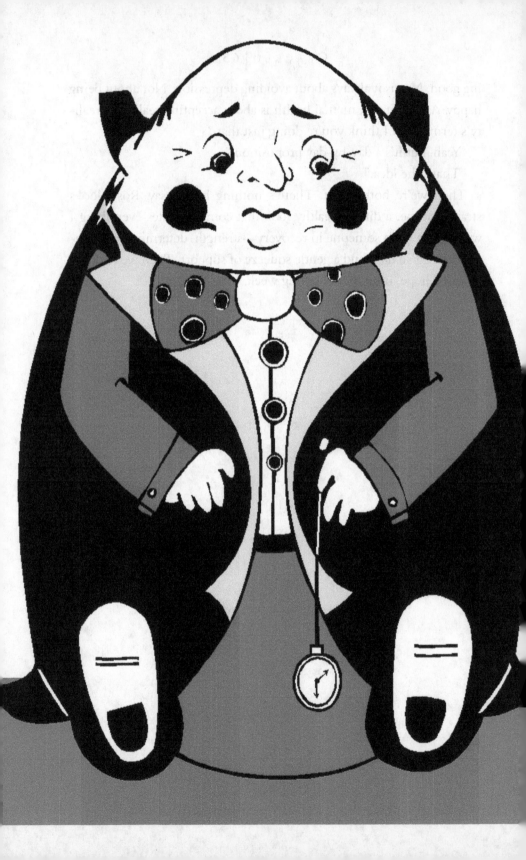

Five

I GET TO the unit at about eleven o'clock, happy to be back. Some days are like that. It simply feels good to be in the corridors, doing the work and going through the routines. The familiarity works for me. I feel connected to something real, as opposed to the chaotic lives of my patients, although today the hallways are empty. In fact, the entire unit is unusually quiet. A counselor tells me that everyone has gone to their groups, following directions as they're supposed to. "Freakish, isn't it?" she muses.

I'm at the nursing station, setting down my briefcase, when Alexi comes in with a cup of coffee.

"I love that one in four-twenty-one," she says.

That's Amber's room. I make her my first stop. She's sitting on the bed, dressed and cleaned up. Her hair is brushed, and there's a hint of color in her face. She hasn't finished detoxing. There'll be many hard times ahead. But for now these are good signs. Leafing through an old *Elle* magazine, she turns to an advertisement for a beauty product and tells me she used to know the girl in the picture. They'd worked together several times as teenage models, but, as Amber explains, they lived on separate coasts and their lives went down separate paths.

"She's making ten G's a day, and I'm here," she says.

"You don't model anymore?" I ask, implying that I think she still could.

"No, not for a long time. I was a kid. It's different now. Like, *duh*. Look at me here."

There are places that could be much worse, but I refrain from saying so. Responding to the intense sugar cravings of early withdrawal, Amber has littered the nightstand with half-eaten Butterfinger and Snickers bars. The floor is strewn with Bobby Brown makeup canisters and undergarments, signs of withdrawal, frustration, and struggle as she tries to write the next chapter in her life. She stares at me with large brown eyes, no longer interested in her magazine.

"You need to start going to groups," I say.

She doesn't pay attention. "I think you're better-looking in person than you are on television."

I take a defensive step backward, then recover, smiling slightly. I'm flattered, but I ignore her flirtation. Hey, I'm not immune to the notion of a very attractive young woman flirting with me. I'm only human. But I know Amber's come-on is a ploy to get what she wants—drugs—using the only tool sexually abused women like her know how to use with men. If it works, she's victimized again. If it doesn't, she's exposed to shame.

Needless to say, she's frustrated. That prompts her to complain angrily about the nursing staff for being unresponsive to her needs.

"In what way are you not being cared for?" I ask.

"I'm in too much pain," she says. "They won't give me any more medication."

"As the doctor responsible for your medical treatment, I know you're getting what you need."

"Then you're doing a shitty job," she says. "I need more. At least something to help me sleep."

"According to the night nurse, you do sleep. It just doesn't feel like it because of your withdrawal."

"Look, I'm serious. You want honest, I'm giving you honest. Here it is: I can get drugs without any problem. Anything I want. Don't make me walk out of here and do something I don't want to do. I can't fuck-ing stand the way I feel, and if I can't get a little help here I'll go else-where."

The look she gives me now is much different than the one a few minutes earlier. I respond by doing nothing and absorbing her anger. Soon she's picking at the frayed ends of her blue jeans.

"This is always a miserable experience," I say. "It's been six days. We're doing everything medically safe to make it tolerable."

"Can't you just put me out till it's over?"

"No. You have to trust that we're doing everything that should be done."

Quiet, she shakes her head. It's easy to read the disgust on her face.

"How can you trust somebody when your own father—"

Pausing, she leans back and reaches over her shoulder to turn off the lamp. I get a good look at her pierced belly button as her short T-shirt hikes up on her stomach. Given her come-on earlier, it strikes me as staged. Her eyes are filling with tears, but she won't let them go. She grabs her teddy bear and strokes one of his legs.

"You know men never say no to me," she says. "I can get anything I want."

"I understand," I reply, getting up from the chair. "But here you'll be hearing no. It's difficult for us to see you suffering. It would be much easier to give you everything you ask for. But it's not about what you want. We say no to your demands because it's what you need."

★ ★ ★

After my rounds, I return to the nursing station and find a piece of paper placed upside down on my chair. I pick it up and turn it over. The top half of the page is a detailed drawing in black ink of a figure in jail, his hands gripping the bars. Beneath that is some writing done in a stylized script that must have taken some time to execute.

Question: Why are you still here?
Answer: I don't fucking know.
Disease: Well, then, let's split. Let's go down guns blazin'.
Me: Get your hands off my throat.
Disease: Then accept me forever.
Me: Relapse is certain. This shit is going to kill me. How far down the rabbit hole must I go?

It's a pretty accurate description of the struggle. I'm wondering which patient might have written this—which of them has shown any artistic ability?—when I hear Alexi raise her voice. This is a woman who doesn't lose control easily. After the hardships of Eastern Europe, as she says, our troubles in the unit are a piece of cake.

That's why it's unsettling to hear her voice carry down the hall like a siren. I race toward the noise. I end up in the doorway to Amber's room. Alexi is leading a significantly larger man out by his wrist, though if he wanted he could shake her off like a gnat. He's about a foot taller than her and maybe a hundred pounds heavier. Like a football player. He looks to be in his early to mid-forties. He's well dressed, in casual sports clothes. Before leaving the room, he turns to Amber and says, "Don't worry, baby. I'll get you what you want."

"This is Amber's husband," says Alexi, looking relieved to see me.

"Jack," he says.

"Dr. Pinsky," I reply. "What's the problem?"

"This nurse isn't helping my wife. Look at her. She's in pain. She's suffering. I can't bear to see it. I don't know how this nurse can just stand there. She needs more medication."

It's not unusual for family members to react this way when seeing loved ones at the height of withdrawal. Understandably, they can't stand seeing them in pain. But of course they don't have any knowledge of the process. Jack's a perfect example. I walk him down the hall, so Amber can't hear the conversation. He's steamed, and I need him to take it down a few notches. Sometimes addicts can intuit what's going on in such situations and use it to their advantage.

"I want to assure you that everything is under control," I say. "Amber is exactly where she's supposed to be."

"She looks a helluva lot worse than when she was strung out at home," he says. "She sounds it, too. I've seen her bad, but never like this. She says she's going to die from the pain."

"You're going to have to trust me," I say. "And you're going to have to trust my staff, whom you can't abuse."

"I'm not a trusting guy," he says sternly.

"But you're going to have to trust me," I say. "She's okay. She's going through withdrawal. It's not easy. She's a pretty sick young woman."

He runs his fingers through his hair and exhales. Suddenly his tone changes and he wants to be my friend, apologizing if he came off too angry. But dealing with Amber has been tough, he says. He's in the hardware business, he explains, the co-owner with his cousin of several hardware stores. He works hard, and he likes to party hard. So did Amber, he says. Poor thing.

"She's hot, though, isn't she?" he says, a comment so inappropriate that I step back in disgust.

I don't like this guy. I don't know if he can tell, but I don't care. I just want to get rid of him.

"Where'd you go to school?" he asks.

"USC for medicine," I say.

"Sorry to hear that," he says. "I played football at Washington. Do I have to say anymore?"

That's my chance, and I seize it. "No, please don't say anymore. I have to get back to work."

Thank goodness he picks up on the cue. I don't know if I could bear talking to him any longer without becoming overtly rude. As he got chummy, my dislike for him grew proportionately. I could tell the type of guy he was, and the sort of relationship he had with Amber. Granted, I'm quick to categorize; it goes with the job. But abused women are attracted to these types—athletes, cops, high-octane men—seeking safety and protection, but getting a severe power imbalance that breaks down into abuse.

As he leaves, Jack laughingly says, "Make her feel better, okay, Doc? I don't want to have to yank her out of this place, too."

After he's gone, I enjoy the silence. I can feel the tension leave my body. Alexi and I share a look of relief. In the nursing station, she's going through the same deep breathing exercise as I am. I shake my head and say, "He could be more difficult to deal with than Amber."

"I can take the borderlines," she says. "But please, don't let their spouses in."

Sometimes my least favorite people are related to the patients I like the most. If I had my way, we'd treat the families alongside the patients. As it is, we do have family sessions several times a week, but they're voluntary. They should be mandatory. I'm positive Jack beats the crap out of Amber, emotionally if not physically. He might do the same to us, too.

I'm doing paperwork in the nursing station when I notice Amber go outside for a smoke and coffee, and I wonder how she was affected by her husband's visit. A few hours have gone by since he left, and she's feeling a need to get outside, something she rarely does. What's that about? I'm feeling protective as well as curious. (What's *that* about? I also wonder.)

Every so often I glance outside to the patio, where there are several old picnic tables, chairs, and ashtrays piled with butts. We try to get the patients to stop smoking, but we are obliged to provide them with a space outdoors where they can indulge their habit. Three patients occupy one table, smoking and continuing a conversation from group. Then there's Amber. Seated by herself, she might as well be in another country. She lights up a Marlboro, takes two puffs, and throws it away. She glances around. I can see she is agitated and unable to concentrate. She gets up and goes back to her room.

I send a nurse to check on her. After some time has passed, I follow up myself. She's on top of her bed, her back against the wall, with a magazine and her teddy bear in her lap. Her eyelids are heavy, but she makes contact. In that instant, I come under her spell—the kind a beautiful woman casts on a man. I want to open the window shade, let in light, and tell Amber she's beautiful.

I don't. But I am so much more human and susceptible than I admit. I tell myself that my vulnerability and openness allow me to appreciate the opportunity I have to make contact, even the most fleeting contact, with someone who's been disconnected from his or her humanity. But part of that, I know, is also BS, an attempt to rationalize my need to rescue.

Amber doesn't care one way or the other. Whatever works for her is good. I know what she wants. "My husband says I should've gone to Cedars," she says. "He says they would've given me more medication."

"Your husband's not a doctor," I respond. "But I am going to change some of your meds. I'm going to give you some Seroquel for your agitation. I'm also going to give you something to help you sleep a little better. But I can't give you anything more to help with the withdrawal."

She reaches for the pink comforter at the end of the bed and pulls it up over her. Is she hiding or cold? Probably both.

"Your husband's a big guy?" I say.

"Yeah. He'll be back."

"Will any other family be coming?"

"You've got to be kidding," she says.

"Not close to them?"

"I love my mom," says Amber. "She's the only one I love."

"What about your father?"

"Fucking freak," she says without hesitation.

As I suspected. This will be helpful for me to hear: The more we know about a patient's background, the better the treatment we're able to provide. Amber isn't very forthcoming, but neither does she refuse to talk. The details come slowly. She grew up middle class in Ontario, a city about sixty miles east of Los Angeles, the younger of two children (her brother's in the military) of a mechanic father and salesclerk mother. She describes a home life that didn't have much structure. There were no regular mealtimes; if she didn't want to go to school, she stayed home in her room.

Most people probably thought they were a nice family, Amber says, but the reality was horrifying. Her father was terribly abusive to her mother. Amber would stand outside the bathroom door and hear everything: the cries, the slaps, the pleading. Things got even worse after Amber told her mother about what her father had been doing to her from age seven on.

"Do you think your mother was sexually abused, too?" I ask.

"She once said something about that," says Amber. "Something about her dad being an alcoholic, too. I don't know. It's all shitty."

The pattern is clear to me. It began with her grandparents, or earlier. Her mother married a man just like her father. Now Amber has done the same. She's just like her mother, thinking she's found a savior when in fact she's just attached herself to a man who is going to repeat the cycle of abuse. I guarantee Jack is that person.

"Does your husband—"

She opens her magazine and looks down at the page. "I don't want to talk anymore," she says in a voice so cold I can feel the room temperature drop.

She's done. The light in her eyes disappears. I glance out the open door, wishing someone would walk in, someone who would stimulate her to talk. This is frustrating for me, pure torture. If I could get her to talk more, I think, I might be able to make the connection she needs. But of course I also think, who needs this more—me or Amber?

Alas, I can't force her to trust me with her innermost thoughts, any more than I can make it rain or snow.

Patients don't have to open up to me or anyone else on staff. There are no rules stipulating that patients must share the details of their lives, the abuses they suffered, their fears, and their mistakes. The mistakes can often be the hardest. I know of a patient who has been in and out of rehab a dozen times over the last decade, and he can't get past the fourth and fifth steps, which require a fearless moral inventory of all one's wrongdoings. It's just too painful.

Of course, some patients can't wait to unload. They'll talk nonstop if we give them the chance. We don't have the time. Others are only comfortable discussing their most painful and private moments among peers or with their sponsors. We emphasize only one thing: The more patients talk honestly about their feelings, the better their chances at recovery.

The opposite is also true. Those who don't talk don't succeed. They don't make connections and grow beyond their old hurts. That's true of the man I mentioned who can't get beyond the fourth and fifth steps. Despite all his treatment, he's never been able to stay sober for more than a few months.

Amber, I can see, is on the fence. She might open up, she might not. I can't tell, and it's too early to make any predictions. She clearly has a lot to say, though. Volumes. I may never learn all or any of the details, but I know enough about the blueprints to make me sick. As a child, Amber was violated by the same grown-ups she loved and believed would give her the nourishment she needed to grow and thrive. Instead she was left helpless, defensive, and struggling to survive. She could never allow herself to trust anyone again, lest it leave her feeling threatened again.

Love? It's not in her vocabulary.

What of her looks, those looks that make men fall in love in a heart-beat? She's been blessed, and yet she can't feel it. Can I make her understand that connecting with others is the only way to help that frightened seven-year-old inside her discover more joy than pain? Will she ever be able to trust enough to take that risk?

For all my training, I can only do so much to treat her, or any addict, for that matter. I can take them through withdrawal. I can administer medications to help them get through detox. But actual long-term recovery is up to them. It's one of the challenges of this type of medicine. A surgeon can put in a new heart or liver and the patient improves. An orthopedist can reset a broken leg and the patient will eventually walk again, whether he works at it or not. But I can't make one of my patients better on my own. I wish I could.

I can provide help while their body chemistry readjusts to a drug-free life. I can talk to them about AA's twelve-step program, encourage them to attend meetings, and arrange for admission into a Sober Living program, where they can receive the structure they need to support their effort to stay clean. I can put in the time and do everything they need to start the healing process. I can be the first real human being they can trust. But that's it.

At a certain point, they just have to want to *get it*.

The light has to go on inside.

The rest of the night passes, and before I know it I'm on my way home from the radio station after three hours of *Loveline* with Adam Carolla. It's close to 1:00 A.M. The freeways are an absolute pleasure to drive when they're this empty. If I weren't so tired, I would enjoy the drive. As I pull into the driveway at home, my beeper goes off. It's the hospital.

I call in and get Diana, the night nurse. Like Alexi, she's wired to remain calm in any situation. She works nights, so I don't see much of her, but Diana and I talk all the time. Her voice never varies in tone. She's always on top of things, quick and efficient. Tonight's emergency is Amber.

"She banged on the medication window for hours," she reports. "She demanded something to help her sleep, and got very frustrated when we said no. She insisted you promised her different meds."

"They were changed," I said. "Alexi took care of that before I left."

"It didn't calm her down. She's been up all night. Agitated. Threatening to leave."

Why the drastic change in her behavior? I believe it's a reaction to the discussion we had. Talking about abuse that way can often open the floodgates to emotions that are difficult to control. At best, she's overwhelmed. Now she's still in an altered chemical state that's got her reeling and confused.

If she wanted to leave, we couldn't do anything to stop her, though we try very hard to talk patients through the situation and hope they stay.

"And now?"

"We worked hard to deescalate her. I had two people stay with her. She hasn't left. That's the best I can say."

"Let's keep it that way," I say. "Thanks for the update."

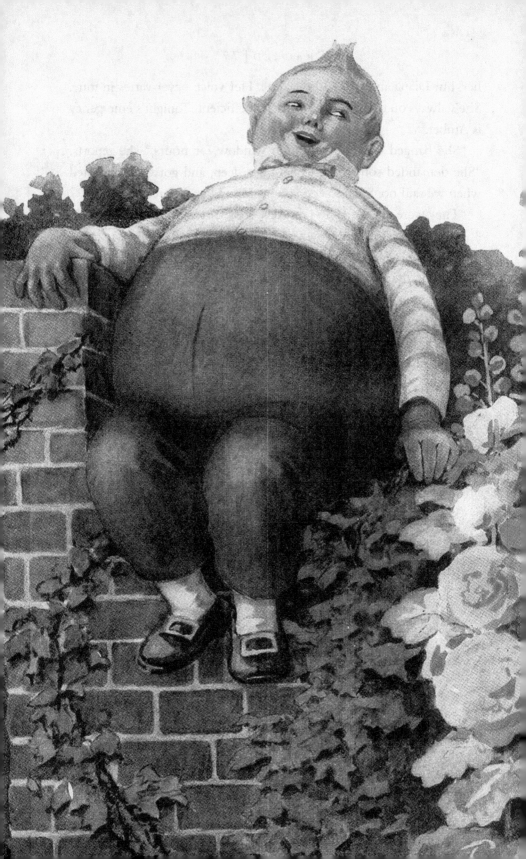

Six

EARLY THE NEXT morning I go online and check my e-mail. Among the junk I find a report informing me that Amber made it through the night, eventually falling into a fitful sleep, and as of 6:00 A.M. she was continuing to rest with her eyes shut. "Still quiet, thank God," the note finishes.

By 10:00 A.M. I'm sitting in the South Pasadena office where I maintain the private practice my father started in the early 1950s. The call is on behalf of Gladys, an elderly patient who began with my dad shortly after I was born. Gladys is fighting a bronchial infection and claims she needs stronger medication. She is one of a few patients I have left who compare me to my father, and usually she gives me good marks.

I do enough comparing on my own. For several years my dad and I worked side by side, the old-fashioned family doctor and his hotshot son fresh out of medical school. It wasn't an easy situation: He struggled to maintain a business-as-usual environment while I scurried around modernizing his office and expanding the number of patients we treated.

There was a time when I thought I wanted to leave my father's practice. After he retired in 1998, though, many of his longtime patients worried out loud that I would abandon them, too. Though I had more lucrative opportunities, I took my commitment to them seriously, and I chose to stay. No regrets here. I enjoy the challenge of diagnosing abnormal biology and figuring out the treatment, and the exposure helps me keep up my skills. Yes, most of my patients are elderly, but old people are the ones who get sick. Anyone who wants to see pathology is going to see an older population. They end up teaching me as much as I help them.

Gladys, my first patient of the morning, is a sixty-seven-year-old grandmother. When I ask how she's been doing, she responds with a deep sigh.

"I almost died this morning when I put on my stockings," she says. "That's how little strength I have."

As I learned from my father, patients often come in simply to talk, and Gladys is one of those. Over the past few years, she has dealt with kidney failure, diabetes, and hypertension. Despite the long list of maladies, she has hung in with impressive resilience. As she says, she doesn't plan on checking out anytime soon. No, she would rather nag. Hence today's appointment. Besides the reassurance that comes from a visit, she wants to know if I agree that her pharmacist is gouging her.

"The charges sound about right," I say, disappointing her. "You can shop around, but you need those pills."

"It's getting so only the rich can afford to get sick or old," she scoffs.

After checking up on several other patients, all routine, I meet Beverly and Richard Norton, a married couple in their mid-eighties. Their visit is a pleasure. He was a successful scrap metal salesman whose winning personality is still evident. Beverly and Richard have a bunch of grandchildren; until recently, they've been avid world travelers. They're adorable, always watching out for each other, always bundled up in sweaters and scarves, even in the summer. They still hold hands. I like them very much.

But Richard is beginning to fail. Age plays no favorites. Beverly is still coughing up sputum. I thought she would be somewhat better, but the stress and fear of what's happening to her husband is taking its toll. After battling heart failure for years, Richard is starting to poop out. His mind is sharp, but his body is simply yielding to age. Richard is exceptional. He seemed to accept the infirmities of aging as a part of life. This sets him apart from most Americans. In this country, we don't care for the aged and diseased. We keep them hidden away in hospitals and institutions, never to dirty our hands with their care, while we inundate ourselves with images of youth and unrealistic messages about optimum health. As a result, most of us are shocked when we age. We expect eternal youth and health. And because we have no sense of our biology, we are bewildered when a medical problem emerges. I'm always amused when a seventy- or eighty-year-old patient with a new medical problem reacts in disbelief. "How could this be? I've never been sick before." The next question is usually, "What did I do to cause this?" Usually, it's just the biological process of aging. And I try to get them to understand that aging beats the alternative.

Addicts in early recovery can be funny this way, too. Soon after they detox, many patients who've spent years killing themselves with alcohol and drugs start worrying over every little symptom. Now that they're waking up and feeling again, every hangnail becomes a potential crisis.

"Dr. Pinsky," Richard says. "I have a question for you."

"Go ahead."

"What do you call an eighty-four-year-old man with a bad heart?"

"I don't know. What?"

"Old."

Richard, always ready with a corny joke or line straight out of the *Saturday Evening Post,* loses his breath laughing at this one. After he recovers, I listen to his chest. His ejection fraction, the percentage of blood pumped out of his heart with each beat, is only 19 percent. It should be around 60. Dip below 20, things aren't good. On previous visits I've suggested that they think about a nursing home, but Richard has always refused, explaining that he's comfortable at home. "I know where the TV clicker is," he always says.

The two of them accepted their health problems a while ago, but Richard's severely weak heart has me very concerned. I suggest checking into a hospital. But he turns me down.

"I'm past worrying about making the grade," he says, coughing. "It's difficult enough getting here. I want to be at home. I like my home."

I hear the subtext of his response and nod, appearing to agree. Then our discussion takes a turn that makes this appointment different from the others. I don't know whether Richard decided ahead of time, but he acknowledges that the end is near, and tells me, "When the time comes, I don't want any machines."

"I understand," I say.

"I want to go out of this world as gently as I came in."

This is a turning point in our relationship as doctor and patient. I want to think our longtime relationship has contributed to this openness. Richard has had a good life, so why shouldn't he attempt the same when he dies? Later, I write out his instructions in his file. If there is any dispute among family members—something I don't expect—such a notation can have the power of a contract. I agree with Richard. As a doctor, I don't believe in sustaining life in a strictly clinical sense. There has to be quality, not just form.

This is the key point in everything I do and believe. My elderly patients constantly reaffirm it. Through them, I have developed a sense about what matters in life. When people have a finite amount of time left, they focus on what's most important, and 99.9 percent of the time it is the same thing—other people. People are not solo acts. Saying "everyone is interconnected" isn't just a cliché. At the end of our lives, it's all about the connections we have made with other people. Filling our memories, they give our lives substance and meaning.

But guess what? Addicts don't make those connections. That ingredient is absent from their lives. They don't connect with other people in ways that create genuine relationships of meaning and depth. Where other people have trust, they have only feelings of fear, hurt, and violation. No matter what's going on in their lives, they are alone, isolated, scared. It is the reason I can say I have seen many people die in peace, but no addicts who live without a lot of pain.

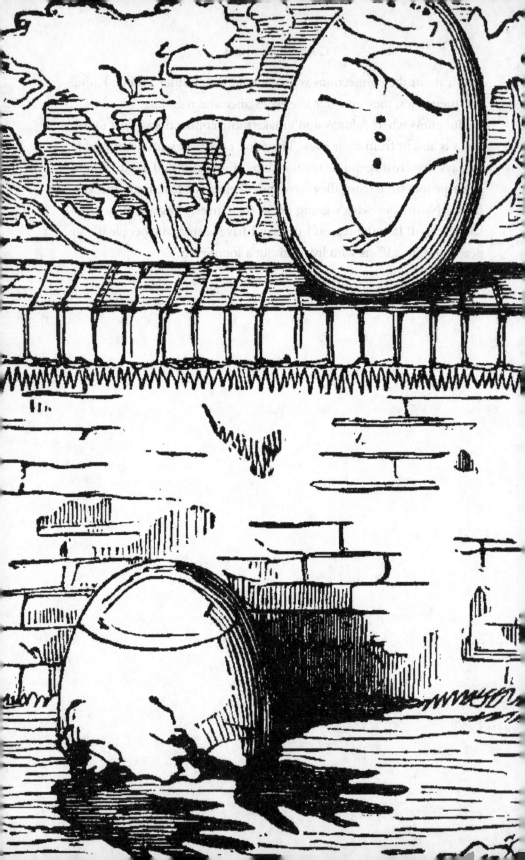

Seven

"HOW IS SHE?" I ask Alexi.

I have been updated on everyone but Amber. I think Alexi purposely saved her for last. She must sense I'm developing a special interest. She liked her instantly, but that was her rising to the challenge of a difficult patient. Now that she's spent more time with Amber, I can tell, she's growing very fond of her.

As in any hospital, we like some patients more than others. At first, we try not to make any judgments. Everyone here is out of it when they first check in, and many are downright miserable from the pain and discomfort. As they come through withdrawal, though, they reveal more of themselves.

Addiction doesn't discriminate. I see every type, from celebrities to bag people. One of my favorite patients was a fundamentalist Christian who managed a religious bookstore and read at Sunday school. Three times a day, she slammed heroin through a tiny vein hidden between her thumb and forefinger. They found her passed out in the bathroom of the bookstore. She was the single most polite person I have ever seen go through withdrawal.

Some patients—no, many patients—are at the other extreme. I see quite a few who are totally despicable. But part of my job is to find something worthwhile about every patient, and even when dealing with the most despicable I have to try to understand the feelings behind the behavior. Generally, the worst-behaved patients are the ones in the most pain. They tend to be people who can't tolerate over-whelming feelings, and when they experience dread, shame, rage, and envy, they project them onto other people.

If I am standing in front of them, they project them onto me. They perceive me as the source and container of their horrible feelings. If you aren't aware of the exchange taking place, they will make you feel horrible. They are great at it. That is their goal. There are others who are capable of being awful, but they have much better skills when it comes to manipulating people, and they make you feel great. Alexi loves these patients. But they're only interested in themselves and their own needs.

Amber is still too profoundly affected by her withdrawal for me to draw any conclusions about her tendencies. Despite her complaints and manipulations, something about this young woman appeals to the staff. Part of it is the way she looks. It's human nature to gravitate toward good-looking people. But Alexi doesn't care about that. She reacts to a more human side that has broken through the storm clouds. Earlier this morning she asked Alexi a few questions that made her seem like a real person.

"I don't like her husband, though," says Alexi.

"I know what you mean," I say. "Is she communicating? Sharing? Saying anything?"

"No. She's in group, but she's still too out of it to even consider doing her first step."

At this stage I'm primarily focused on the biological grip the patient is in, but I also try to start educating them about how that relates to the powerlessness of their addiction. The messages are direct. We introduce the ideas of the twelve steps, powerlessness, and the behavioral goals we want them to achieve. We repeat these things over and over, since in the delirium of withdrawal very little sticks.

Then again, I don't know what makes patients admit they're powerless over their addiction.

I don't know what makes a patient stop using.

Or what finally makes them *get it.*

I have searched long and hard for the answer. I don't think anyone knows, those in AA with longtime sobriety included. A particular woman comes to mind. She had struggled through three previous hospitalizations during which she never made any progress. As soon as she left, she relapsed. But this latest admission was very different. She was attending groups, participating actively, and following directions. Then, at my weekly medical lecture, she suddenly stood up as I was discussing the biology of addiction and said she had something to share.

"I heard you go over all this biology stuff that last time I was here," she said. "But I didn't get it. I just want you and everyone else to know that now I feel completely different about everything you're telling us. Now I get it." She hit her head. "The message got through my thick skull. I get it. But let me ask you a question. What took so long? How do you give someone *'get it'?*"

The room was quiet, and I could feel the room turn its attention from her back toward me. I was suddenly at a loss. I didn't know what to say. I was dazzled by the simplicity and clarity of her question. After all, it was *the* question every addict has to address. The same with me. I think about it with every single patient. How can I make him or her get it?

How do you get people to follow directions, make connections, and trust when they've never done it before?

How do you make them understand that they didn't deserve the abuse they suffered as children?

How do you make them whole again?

It is a complex and mysterious process, so much so that most of my patients who get it attribute it to divine intervention. They say God steps into their lives, which explains the spiritual component of recovery.

"You want to know how to give someone 'get it'?" I asked.

"Yeah," she said.

"Well, if you figure that one out, let me know. We'll bottle it and share the Nobel Prize."

Here's the truth I tell my patients: I don't always have the answer. It drives me nuts. I have no idea why some people get it and others don't. You can't bet on anyone. Those who seem like sure bets often relapse, and those who you think are going to walk out and score sometimes get sober for the rest of their life. Take another former patient, Nancy, a forty-eight-year-old biker living in the high desert. She was a longtime speed and heroin addict who was close to death when paramedics brought her into the unit.

I remember telling Alexi that she wasn't going to make it. Then, when it looked like she would survive, I figured she'd split as soon as she detoxed, and start using again at home. Actually, I suspected the only reason she had checked in in the first place was to escape her abusive, morphine-addicted Vietnam vet boyfriend.

She made it through treatment, but then I heard nothing from her for a year and a half. Then one day I walked into the unit, and she was there. I didn't recognize her. She looked great. I thought she was a visitor; then I did a double-take and realized who she was. After treatment, she had gone through Sober Living for a few months, left her boyfriend, and started over. I asked all sorts of questions. From her answers, I could tell she'd found a way to do it: She was managing her feelings without feeling overwhelmed, or giving in and getting high. She was making one healthy decision after another. The way she described it, her new life was happening almost spontaneously, as if she couldn't help it.

"What happened?" I asked. "What made the difference?"

"I don't know," she said. "I just got it."

Amber could have the same thing. The turning point could come at any time. There's no way I can predict what could be the catalyst. But when Alexi and I stop in her room during our rounds, my first thought is not positive. She gives me the impression it might take a bomb exploding beneath her to snap her into a state resembling consciousness. She's lying on her bed in jeans and a T-shirt cropped below her breasts. It's so short my instinct is to turn away. She looks wasted, and she is. Her body chemistry is still a mess from the drugs she's coming down from, and from the meds we're giving her.

Alexi hangs by the door. I pull a chair next to her bed and sit down. "How's it going?" I ask.

"I still feel like shit."

"It's going to be a while," I say.

Our conversation is run-of-the-mill. Amber doesn't have any significant memory of her first few days in treatment. She doesn't remember whether she has slept. "It doesn't feel like it," she says, repositioning herself on the bed with a long, slow groan that sounds like it has worked through her entire body. "God, I hate this," she adds, before telling me she doesn't recall her constant demands for more drugs or complaints about being mistreated by the staff. She has attended groups, where she has taken the same seat in the back each time, but she hasn't participated. She hasn't done any work.

There's a magazine beside her. *Vogue.* I pick it up, riffle through the pages, and set it back down.

"Anything interesting in here?" I ask.

"I don't know," she says. "I don't have the energy to look. I'm not sleeping. I could use some better sleepers."

She has already picked up the jargon for nighttime pills. It doesn't take long before patients start sounding like residents, throwing around the lingo: *sleepers, meds, benzos.* Like good addicts, they might not be able to keep track of meals and meetings, but within minutes they sound as if they've memorized the *Physicians' Desk Reference.*

"You're getting all the medication you can take safely."

Amber shuts her eyes. Moments pass.

"I feel like crap. When's this going to be over?" she sighs.

I slowly describe the process of withdrawal, treatment, Sober Living, and long-term recovery. Rather than think about a lifetime of sobriety, I urge her to concentrate on one day at a time. She has to make herself whole again, and that's a long, slow, often painful progression of baby steps. Amber rolls her eyes. She wants me to give her drugs. Nothing else will satisfy her.

"I know you don't trust anyone," I say. "And I know you don't have any faith. But those are the two things you need."

"How can I trust?" she says, her voice tinged with disbelief and scorn. "What do you know about trust? My father raped me when I was seven. I've had the crap beat out of me so many times." Her voice trails off. "My husband—"

Amber closes her eyes and tears slide down her face. My stomach tightens. I can feel her misery crawling under my skin. I wish it weren't so, but I can't help it. The more Amber makes her awful feelings tangible and real, the more I feel them, too. Patients think they go through it alone. They don't. Why do you think there's so much stress on caregivers? Doctors and nurses, too. Bill Clinton gave the phrase "I feel your pain" a bad name, but we doctors do. It's inescapable. It is the toughest part of treatment for me, the most draining, and yet it's also the part I connect with, the part that makes me feel like a rescuer.

My job isn't to rescue anyone, though. My job is to help Amber help herself. Am I doing that as best I can? I don't know. That sort of awareness is lost in the moment.

"I'd be better off dead," she says.

"I know why you say that," I reply. "But no one your age is better off dead."

"Then what can you do for me?" she asks.

"I'm doing everything I can. You have to pitch in, too."

"I just want to go to sleep. Or, like, get the hell out of this place."

"You can get better. I see it happen over and over to people who feel a lot worse than you. You have to have faith."

She rolls over and faces the wall. "Yeah. Right."

I exhale and glance back at Alexi, who knows but doesn't share my frustration. She finds it easier to accept the process the patient goes through. She goes with the current. She waits for openings, and finds amusement when there are none. I have to work at it a lot harder. Conclusions like this one leave me unsatisfied, angry, feeling as if I haven't done all that I can. Not that I can do anything about it. I can't magically change the patient, though I wish I could. I wish Amber would respond in a way that made me feel better. The rescuer in me wants results that make me feel good. But that's my problem, not hers.

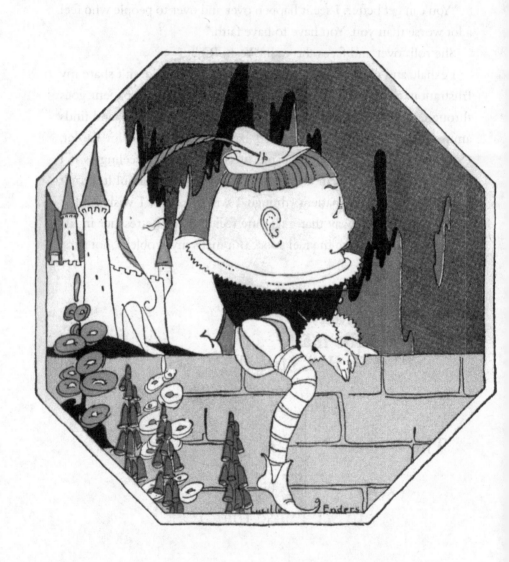

Eight

LOS ANGELES HAS two distinct flavors. By day, it's a sprawling metropolis by the ocean. No matter how far inland you go, the city is still defined by the surf, sand, and sunshine. At night, it is a completely different story. The vibe is neon and nasty. With the lights on, you hear the Beach Boys and think about Hollywood. When the lights are off, you hear Jim Morrison and the Doors and think about Heidi Fleiss.

My life changes after dark, too. Five nights a week, between 10:00 P.M. and midnight, I take on the role of Dr. Drew, the co-host of *Loveline,* a syndicated call-in radio program where young people—the curious, the disenfranchised, the stoners, and the kooks—phone in with questions about sex, drugs, and everything in between. About four hours after leaving Amber, I arrive at the Westwood One radio complex where the show is broadcast. My co-host, Adam Carolla, shows up a few minutes later. By then the studio is abuzz with activity as our producers line up phone callers.

"No way! You're lying," I hear Brad, one of the screeners, tell a caller before breaking into a full-on laugh. Soon the other screener is laughing, and then one of the producers joins in.

"What's going on?" I ask.

Brad puts the caller on hold and explains: For the past couple of years, the caller claims, he's been acting on an unusual compulsion.

"What's that?" I ask.

"He says he eats dog poop."

"Yeah?"

"He wants to know if that's weird. And if he can get sick."

"That's a fake," I say, though I give the caller credit for being funny, in a twisted sort of way.

"Hey, man," says Brad. "I don't know about your call. You might be goofing on us. If you aren't, try calling a vet."

It's one of the few calls we don't take on *Loveline*. One of the things I love about doing the show is our no-holds-barred policy. Our job is to give information, not pass judgment. Callers can ask whatever they want, and they do, every night we go on the air. If a kid has a question about the workings of a penis or a vagina, this is the place to call. If a kid has never talked to anyone about an orgasm, *Loveline* can help. If they've tried pot and want to know what it does to them, or they're curious about Ecstasy, they can call the show and find out the truth. The program has created a community, a place where healthy dialogue can lead listeners to healthy decisions. If those decisions lead to healthier lives, then I'm doing my job as a doctor.

The show is one of the things I am proudest of, but it was a happy accident. In 1983, KROQ, a small FM station in Pasadena, was redefining pop music by playing the Sex Pistols, the Clash, and Elvis Costello, then cutting-edge artists taking over from the well-worn 1970s acts like Led Zeppelin, Van Halen, and Foreigner who'd gone before.

As the station took off, the program director, himself an addict, was looking to put a community service show on the air, and he assigned two of his wilder DJs, the Swedish Eagle and the Poorman, to create one in the midnight-to-3:00 A.M. slot on Sundays. These were talented, creative guys who designed a call-in show around the topics they talked about all the time—sex and drugs—figuring listeners would be interested in the same thing. Then, to give it at least a taste of public service, they came up with the idea of a regular segment called "Ask a Surgeon." All they needed was the surgeon.

A mutual friend recommended me. I was no surgeon, of course, just a medical student. But Eagle and Poorman didn't care. "We just want you to use big words," they explained. I declined, thinking they were too silly for someone as serious-minded as myself, but they persisted. We had a very weird meeting at our friend's apartment, during which Poorman, in a terry-cloth vest and shorts nodded off in midsentence after we were introduced. Later, he had me discuss the show while he took a shower.

After all was said and done, I told him I still didn't get it.

"Dude, don't worry about it," he replied. "Just show up."

By the next day, the guys were on the air promoting the new show and promising there would be a real doctor talking about VD and other cool stuff. That weekend, I appeared on *Loveline* for the first time. Listeners couldn't talk enough about sex and relationships and drugs. They had a million questions. The show took off.

Despite my naiveté, I realized what I'd stumbled into: the chance to do something unique by talking to young people, to give them the facts they needed and couldn't get elsewhere. The average listener, fifteen to eighteen years old, was starved for honest information. AIDS was still known as GRIDS (Gay Related Intestinal Disease Syndrome). The phrase "safe sex" hadn't been coined. Condoms were still sold from behind the pharmacist's counter. Dr. Ruth had just emerged, offering her own brand of frank talk about sex, but she didn't have much credibility among kids, or knowledge of the medical consequences of their behavior. And as for drug use, it just wasn't discussed. "Just say no" was all there was to say. It was a joke.

I was only twenty-four. I didn't preach or moralize. I didn't tell anyone not to do drugs, or to abstain from sex. I *couldn't*, without sounding like a parent, and I certainly wasn't anyone's parent. I knew I would be most effective simply by providing facts and explaining the consequences. Straight up.

Not everyone agreed. I didn't go looking for publicity. That wasn't my thing. But after an article about the show was printed in the *Los Angeles Times* in 1985, the doctor supervising my internship at Huntington Memorial Hospital, a brilliant man who specialized in liver disease, gave me a dressing-down for going on the radio and acting in what he considered an unprofessional manner. Devastated, for the first time I found myself doubting something I knew was right and good.

Worried that my future might be in jeopardy, I took a six-month break from the show, and during that period I noticed a shift in the culture. A new openness began emerging about the very subjects I'd been talking about on the radio. Suddenly everyone seemed to be discussing things like safe sex and condoms. They were now seen as legitimate concerns. Vindicated, I went back on the radio. And best of all, three years later the doctor who had reprimanded me asked whether I'd consider stepping aside—to let him take over.

Adam and I are opposites. We get along, and somehow we share the same sensibility. But we're very different. As he once told the *Los Angeles Times*, "When Drew was nineteen, he was premed at Amherst. When I was nineteen, I was cleaning carpets out by Edwards Air Force Base at three in the morning and hanging out with a scary guy named Everlastin' who smoked a joint while driving our van at ninety-five miles per hour."

You can hear the difference, too. Adam is funny. He'll say anything. I try to be a little saner, always authoritative, and usually appropriate. Our first caller this evening brings that out. She's in her early twenties, and she asks a question that reminds me that we're still filling a vital need two decades after *Loveline* debuted.

"Is anal sex related to respect?" she asks. "I mean, my boyfriend wants to do it, and I agreed."

"You already did it, right?" says Adam.

"Yeah," she admits.

"This issue of respect you mentioned," I cut in. "Does your boyfriend abuse you?"

She's silent. Adam prods her for a response.

"Yes, uh-huh," she says reluctantly. "Sometimes."

"Was your father an alcoholic?" I ask.

"Uh-huh."

"Did he hit your mother?"

"Yes."

"Did he abuse you?"

"He didn't hit me, but . . . you know, like any kid, when I was bad . . . "

"Do you and your boyfriend get high?" I ask.

"Yes."

"Does he drink?"

"Uh-huh."

"Is that when he hits you?"

"Uh-huh."

"Sounds like a party to me," Adam chimes in.

"It's not a party, though," I say. "Your boyfriend is like your father, and you're playing the role of victim, which you've played your whole life. You've cast your play perfectly."

"Drew, I'd say your performance with this caller is outstanding," cracks Adam, trying to lighten the moment.

"I know you called about something else," I continue, "but you know what? You need help. You need treatment. You need to make different, healthier choices in your life."

"Yeah, I guess," she says.

"The pattern of repeating is not unusual," I say, wrapping up. "It's normal. It's a kind of compulsive destructive thing. If you're totally honest right now, I bet you'll admit the little voice in your head has often said, 'Not this guy again.' "

Eight more calls are waiting to get on the air. On average, we'll talk to fifteen or twenty people a show. Men typically phone in with sex-related questions, usually about adequacy and performance. They want to know if they're normal. Women are more interested in relationships. They also ask about the way men's minds work. Why does he want a threesome? How come he likes lesbians?

But the calls run the gamut. They're entirely unpredictable.

"Hi, I cut myself with a rusty knife this morning and now my arm is red and it hurts real bad," says the next caller. "Should I go to the hospital?"

"Have you heard of flesh-eating bacteria?" asks Adam. "You moron. Of course you should go to the hospital."

"Yeah, get it checked," I concur.

No questions are stupid to us. There's no problem too small or weird or way out. Anyone who thinks otherwise has only to imagine a kid twenty years ago asking about "that new gay sex disease." Those who criticize the show for being too graphic don't get it. They need to ask why the language is real and direct. There's a drama behind every question. There are other Ambers are out there, and often we're the only people they can speak to openly and without fear.

Never underestimate the power of the airwaves. I remember being interviewed in Portland, Oregon, by a reporter whose questions were unusually perceptive. As soon as his show ended I asked him a few questions, and he confessed he'd been a heroin addict on the streets, turning tricks to maintain his habit. I wasn't surprised. He said he'd been sodomized as a kid by his minister father, who screamed epithets from the Bible as he raped his son.

His story made me ill, but he wasn't telling me all that to make me feel bad. The opposite was true. He said that when he was on the streets he and his gang of teenage homeless prostitute friends would gather around the radio and listen to *Loveline,* and for whatever reason he allowed himself to connect with me. It was the first time he believed an adult could actually care about a kid.

Motivated to get help, he went to the department of psychiatry at the local university, got a referral, and saw a therapist every day for years. Describing the pain of those sessions, he said, "Sometimes I wanted to fuck my therapist, other times I wanted to kill him. But I couldn't stand it if I was away from him."

The show also affected his friends deeply. According to him, many of them couldn't tolerate listening to an entire show. If Adam or I were connecting with a particularly poignant or disturbed caller, they'd drift away from the radio, literally walking away. They couldn't handle the raw emotions coming through the radio. They were connecting that strongly. It was as though the thought of a caring adult reminded them of how differently they'd been dealt with by adults. It was too painful.

"Let's take another call," says Adam. "Neal, you're twenty years old. What's up?"

"My girlfriend and I have trouble having sex," the caller says.

"What kind of trouble?" I ask.

"I can't do it unless I'm watching porn," he says.

"Unless you're paying the thirteen-fifty they charge at hotels, I don't see the problem," Adam says. "Drew, why don't you handle this?"

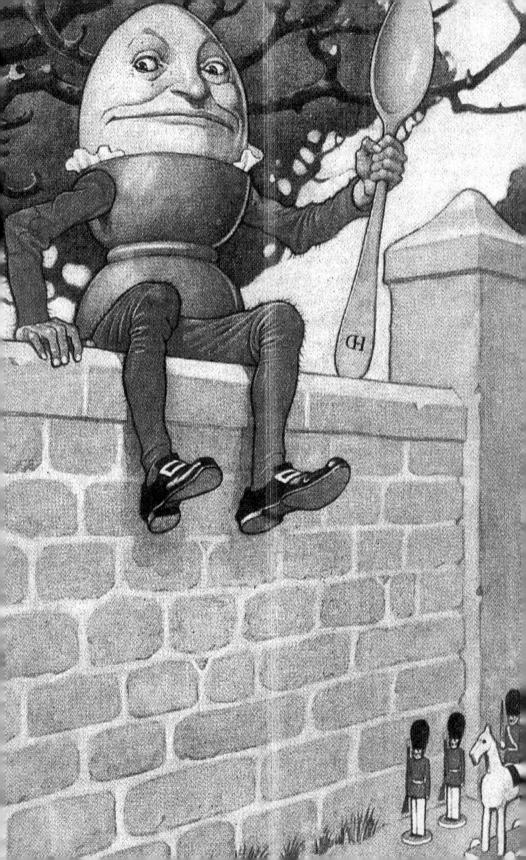

Nine

AFTER TWO DAYS off from the unit, I come back and find out there's good news about Amber. Now in her tenth day of treatment, she has participated in several groups and socialized with her peers out on the patio. She's not exactly born again, but that's not the way it works. Recovery is slow, incremental, and often imperceptible, like watching the grass grow. But at least the news is positive. That's a pretty good way to start the day. But then Alexi seems unsure about letting me feel too upbeat.

"She still has her not-so-good moments," she cautions.

"Don't look so happy," I say.

"If we could just get rid of her pain-in-the-ass husband, she might make a little more progress. She doesn't react well after his visits."

"When was he here?"

"Last night."

"Do you think he's bringing in drugs?"

"No, but we do need to keep an eye on him."

After lunch, I spot Amber on the patio, soaking up some sun. She's wearing silk pajamas that reveal too much skin. I ask Alexi to go out and get her to put on some decent clothes. No wonder she's so popular with the male patients. Later, Alexi trails behind me as we enter Amber's room. The floor is strewn with clothes. Amber has put on a baggy sweatshirt over her pajamas.

"How are you feeling?" I ask.

"How do you think I feel?" she says. "I want to get high. I just keep thinking about running out of here. But don't freak. I'm not going to."

"Listen, you've come this far. We can get you through this. It's going to get better over the next couple of days. Going to group—"

I'm about to advise her to use group as a motivator, as a way to help get her mind off how bad she feels, when she interrupts me. "I'm going to group, but today *PAT* "—one of our counselors—"kicked me out."

I glance at Alexi. "She was too disruptive," she explains.

"Has anyone talked to you about doing a first step?" I ask.

"You've got to give me something for this diarrhea I have," she says. "I shit on myself this morning."

"Alexi, add Imodium. Two with each loose stool. Up to eight per day."

There's only so much I can do for the diarrhea from oral opiate withdrawal. And treating it often perpetuates the problem.

"Did Pat give her the first-step material?" I ask Alexi. She just stares at me.

I move closer to Amber and examine her heart and lungs. Her breathing sounds coarse.

"Are you smoking?" I ask.

"Everyone smokes in this place," she says. "I hadn't smoked in years." She turns away from me and looks at Alexi. "I need some more of that phenobarb. I have two blown discs in my back, and I need something for the pain."

I don't know anyone who doesn't have back pain. It's our heritage from having come off all fours. But Amber's pain isn't from blown discs. I guarantee it. She is suffering from opiate withdrawal. She needs that repeated over and over, which is okay with me. I have those lines memorized.

"You have at least four reasons for back pain," I say. "First, you probably have some disc problem that causes pain. But that discomfort would be tolerable if your brain's endogenous morphine system weren't so severely altered by all the pain meds you've been taking for years. Second, withdrawal from these causes crushing back pain.

"Third, you were severely abused. Abuse victims often complain of pelvic and back pain. It's like your body is trying to tell us your story when you have no other way to express your pain.

"And finally, of course, there is your disease. People with addicted brains learn that if they have pain they get the reward their brain so desperately seeks. You are powerless over this mechanism. This is the first principle we want you to get your head around. Maybe we could get you the first-step material so you can begin to look at how this has made your life so chaotic and unmanageable."

Without missing a beat, Amber says, "Okay, but what can I have for the back pain?" She looks to Alexi for an answer.

"You're not going to cut back that phenobarb, are you?" she continues. "I heard someone on the patio say that you brought me down too fast."

"Not true," I say. "Let us worry about your treatment." I turn to Alexi and give instructions that should help with the withdrawal pain. "Let's D.C. the Motrin and begin Toradol thirty milligrams IM every eight."

I am done. I signal Alexi, who can't wait to get out of the room. We confer in the hall.

"Why are you wasting your time with trying to get her to do the first step?" Alexi asks. "You know she won't remember any of this."

She is right. Amber is too caught up in her own world to deal with the information I gave her. She wants one thing. Her addicted brain can't get beyond the craving for drugs. She is gripped in that vise, and there's no room in her head for anything else. Many experience amnesia early in treatment from the biological effects of withdrawal and the meds we give them to treat it. I don't know why I kept talking to her as if she understood.

Actually, I do. I couldn't help myself.

The rest of the day is uneventful, until Alexi asks me to help with a new patient in Room 257.

Linsey is on the bed, staring out the window. At first glance, she doesn't appear to be trouble. She is twenty-eight, skinny, with a round face and short brown hair. Her left nostril is decorated with a thin gold ring. She had OD'd the day before, and spent the night in a South Bay hospital. Her mother brought her to Las Encinas this afternoon. As soon as I enter, Linsey makes eye contact and starts in on her symptoms.

"It hurts right here," she says, rubbing the middle of her chest.

I take out my stethoscope and listen to her chest.

"It's likely you had an overzealous paramedic, who got carried away with his CPR," I say, continuing the exam.

Extremely agitated, Linsey rubs her arms and thighs and scratches at her calves as if she is trying to peel off several layers of skin. She might if she doesn't stop. But she can't. Several times I have to ask her to be still so I can continue the exam. She apologizes and sits on her hands, which stops the scratching for a few seconds, but then the poor girl starts up again, completely unaware that she can't control herself. I don't find any track marks on Linsey. Her nasal septum is intact. Her lungs are clear. She doesn't have any murmurs. Neither does she have any scars from cutting or picking. Her hair isn't banded. In fact, she appears to be in remarkably good shape.

While examining her head and neck I notice something I often find with my patients, fullness at the angle of her jaw just in front of her ear.

"Have you ever noticed this?" I ask.

Linsey rubs her finger over the spot. She feels the fullness.

"No, never," she says, shaking her head. "What is it? Is it cancer?"

"No, it's not cancer," I say.

Her parotid or salivary gland is swollen. I don't know whether it's from chronic marijuana use, alcohol, or the effects of an eating disorder, but I find this in so many patients that it often provides a more accurate history than what the patient tells me. I take another look at her chart and reread the toxicology report. It turned up benzodiazepines, opiates, alcohol, and three different antidepressants. Nice job.

Time for a little conversation. Linsey, I learn, is an accomplished graphic artist from the 90210 zip code. She describes her upbringing as the dark side of the golden ghetto. She was twelve when her alcoholic father and "schizy" mother got divorced. That same year she began smoking pot. By fourteen, she was bulimic. In response, she was sent to boarding school in Colorado. She felt profoundly abandoned. The summer before her senior year she decided to get even with her parents by doing any drug she could get—coke, heroin, speed. Several times she prostituted herself out to friends for drugs.

When her parents found out about their daughter's massive drug problem, they put her in treatment. She bounced from one facility to another as if she were touring colleges. According to Linsey, she's spent time in Minnesota, Arizona, and several L.A. rehabs. But six months is the longest she's ever stayed clean on her own, though before this most recent binge she put together nine sober months by attaching herself to another addict. They mistakenly believed that they helped each other stay clean, but when that relationship ended so did her sobriety.

"What were you taking yesterday when you OD'd?" I ask.

"I don't remember," she says. "All I know is that I woke up in the hospital yesterday."

"Is that why you're here?"

"No," she says. "I'm here because I'm fucked up."

I don't write that down. She can see by my lack of reaction that she hadn't given me enough. This is not an assembly line. Treatment isn't like a bad public school, where students are passed to the next grade just for showing up.

If Linsey is going to get better, she has to start with something real. I don't want to hear the standard lines: "I got tired of living like this." "My life is screwed up." Something profound must have happened to get her into treatment. I want to her to tell me about that. That's the best starting place.

I warn her that she's going to go through withdrawal. I tell her some of the things she should expect and assure her that we'll do everything within our power to keep her comfortable.

"You're going to feel pretty lousy," I say. "But tell Alexi all of your symptoms."

"Okay," she says.

Once Alexi and I are alone, she raises a red flag. She thinks Linsey is withholding details about recent use. She predicts trouble. I blow some hot air into my fist and prescribe a protocol of medication that should help get Linsey through the discomfort she's going to experience over the following week.

After twenty years of treating addicts, I've learned not to expect anything. Every time I have felt as if I have someone figured out, they surprise me. It never fails, for better or for worse. I have become so used to being lied to by my patients. We have a saying: "If their lips are moving, they're lying." We just lost a young nurse who seemed to be doing well in treatment—or so I thought. It turned out she was continuing to chip heroin. Her peers found her dead at home when she didn't show up for her meetings. This disease can be cunning as well as baffling.

At the end of the day, Amber is visited by her husband again. I'm not aware of it until I hear him badgering the nurses outside his wife's room for medication. He insists that Amber is supposed to be getting more phenobarbital for back pain, and invokes my name when the staff doesn't comply. That doesn't work, either, which instigates a belligerent tirade that rattles the hallways and escalates a handful of patients, including his wife.

The nurse who finds me describes the man causing the disturbance as a "pain in the ass," and right away I know who it is. I hurry to the med window. Amber's husband is still carrying on. He stops yelling upon seeing me. Rather than feel embarrassed, he thinks I'm going to help him. I see the way he suddenly changes. I can tell what he's thinking: *Finally, the guy in charge.* He sidles up to me and puts an arm on my shoulder. I step aside, putting a little distance between us.

This guy may think he's trying to help his wife, but he's more the problem than the solution. Not that he could see that for himself, of course. "Drew, I'm glad you're here," he says. "My wife is in pain. Amber is suffering real bad."

"We're doing everything we can for her," I say. "You have to trust us. We know what to do."

"But I just saw her and she's not doing well," he says. "I mean, we could do this at home. She could be in bed there."

"I think this is the best place for her," I say, leading him away from the nursing station and down the hall. I glance over my shoulder toward the nursing station and see Alexi and some of the others applauding in silence and giving me a thumbs-up sign. The nurses don't deserve such treatment from anyone. Nor do they have time.

We stop outside Amber's room. I look in and see that she is calm. She can afford to be calm. She has her husband acting out for her. She thinks he's going to score.

"What's going on?" I ask.

"Look, Amber is driving me crazy," he says. "I know she's a pain in the ass, but it kills me to see her like this."

I reassure him that she's okay. She's doing fine. Her pain is completely normal. So is her desperation for relief.

"Can't you just give her some more of that barbital and maybe just make her sleep?"

"She's having a very intense withdrawal," I say. "We're giving her everything that we can safely."

He takes a moment to digest this information. Then he shakes his head. All of a sudden he acts very chummy. "I've never had to deal with anything like this before," he says.

"I know it's tough to understand, but what you need to do is let us take care of her. These nurses know what they're doing. They've done thousands of detoxes. What you need to do is go to family groups and look into Al-Anon.

"If she's going to have a successful recovery, you're going to have to change as well. I know you're eager to get her back the way she was before the drug use really took off, but that is simply not possible. She has some real serious problems here, and she's going to have work very hard at growing and changing."

Hoping to get through to Jack enough that he'll get off her back and maybe even start taking a look at his own problems, I take a stab at educating him. "I think a simple way to think of relationships is like a lock and key. Emotionally, when two people come together they fit together in much the way the jagged edge of a key fits with the tumblers of a lock. But any traumatic emotional change can change the way those tumblers are shaped.

"That's what happens when a drug addict starts coming to terms with her problems—and it can be very scary to be involved with someone who's going through those emotional changes. It can be very uncomfortable when you no longer fit the way you always did. It can feel like you're losing your partner. Most people instinctively try to force the relationship back to the old familiar territory, but that's usually very bad for someone struggling with recovery. Think of the lock and key again: If the lock changes, the key will have to be changed as well if it's going to continue to fit. Forcing a key into a lock, after all, usually breaks the lock.

"She has no choice, Jack. Her survival depends upon making change. It's your job to keep up with her. And having the important people in an addict's life participate in codependency recovery programs like Al-Anon has a profoundly positive impact on how a patient will do in treatment."

I'm not sure he's really registered what I'm saying, though. "My brothers and I, we all grew up on a farm in Washington State. We went to college, but my dad and my grandfather were farmers. They taught us that if we had a problem, we had to grit it out. Just suck it up. You're like us, educated. So you know, if you apply your mind to something, you can get through it. Amber doesn't know anything about that."

I take a deep breath, and try to answer this. "But I have to tell you, there are certain problems in humans that can't be solved by sheer grit alone. Addiction is one of them. It involves changing some of the noncognitive parts of the brain. And that takes time. It also takes *you* making some changes along with her."

Jack puts his hand on my shoulder.

"Just see if you can give her something more. There must be a way you can make her comfortable."

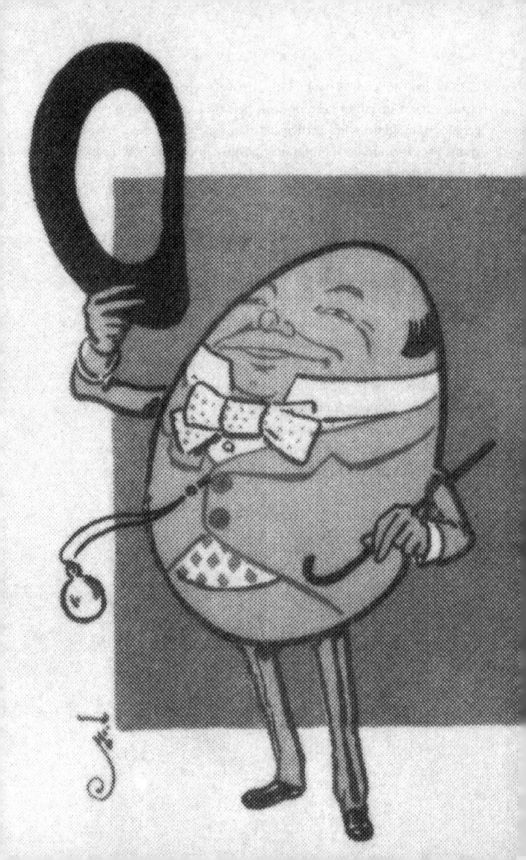

Ten

WHEN I ARRIVE home, I find my wife on the back-door steps, looking through a photo album. It's a warm night, the air as comfortable as a light blanket. Through the glare of city lights, the sky is full of stars. I sit down beside Susan, close enough to see over her shoulder. She flips through the pages, searching for something, and then hands me a yellowed piece of paper that has several folds where it is also starting to tear.

"What's this?" I ask.

"Just look."

It's a prescription written many years ago by her grandmother Marie's brother, Rajvik, a doctor in Prague.

"Cool. What's up with this?"

She reminds me of the psychic party she hosted the previous night for her friends. "The psychic mentioned Prague *and* Rajvik. Then today I found this."

We go inside the house and page through several more family albums. It turns into a night of remembering Marie. Susan's grandmother was twelve when she emigrated to the United States from Prague to escape the Nazis. She married in her early twenties and settled in Cleveland, where she and her husband ran a family restaurant and raised two boys. After her husband died at fifty-two, she continued running the restaurant for years, remaining active—even in the archery club—until she died at ninety-two. Never wealthy, she led a rich and enviable life thanks to a lifetime of interests, activity, and friendships.

Susan and I spend some time sharing our hopes that our lives can be as full and as rewarding as her grandmother's. We dated for years when we were young, then broke up briefly because I wasn't ready to settle down. Then we got back together, and we've been happily married since 1991. We have triplets. Between work, friends, school, lessons, sports, and everything else, we squeeze as much into each day as possible. Any more and both of us would probably live on the freeway. As it is, our cars are like rolling apartments or offices, with all the crap we throw into the backseats.

The lives we lead today are longer than those of our parents, but more hectic. I can't imagine the world my kids, Douglas, Jordan, and Paulina, will inherit when they are my age. It frightens me. Our culture is just like the junk food we live on: It fills you up without the distracting burden of nourishment. An average person exposed to television, movies, and magazines is overwhelmed by messages that arouse, stimulate, and suggest that the answer to all problems is the same: *gratification*. Have a beer, take a pill, roll on the deodorant, get a Whopper, JUST DO IT!

These are just diversions from an empty world. If you've been abused, if you don't know how to trust, and if you're already overwhelmed by feelings you can't handle, an icy six pack won't solve anything. Nor will a new pair of Nikes. Nor will ninety-nine new ways to drive your man wild in bed, as all the women's magazines promise. They aggravate the situation. They ignore the problems. Sadly, the culture offers few messages that address what it means to be human, how to go about feeling healthy. We forget that people feel best when they're interacting, talking, helping, and creating with other people.

"Are you still going tomorrow?" Susan asks. I'm scheduled to take an overnight trip to New Jersey for a speaking engagement at Princeton University.

"Yes," I say. "My flight is early."

The next evening I am in front of 750 students. I do several such talks each month at high schools and colleges. I generally open by talking about the lessons I've learned from my own life. I tell my audiences to listen to their instincts, to that inner voice that has an opinion on everything you do. I don't think the importance of instincts, let alone how to hear them or follow them, is emphasized enough in our children's education.

"If you live your life with integrity, with a clear sense of right and wrong, you will hear that voice more clearly," I say. "It tells you who you should be dating, what you should be doing with your life, when something doesn't feel right, and when you feel good. And it's usually correct."

From there it's an easy step into a discussion about interpersonal relationships, the meat and potatoes of my talk. They know me from *Loveline,* and they expect to hear me talk about sex and drugs, men and women, the whole gestalt of their world when their noses aren't pressed into books. To them, life is supposed to resemble a beer commercial or MTV's spring break beach house. They are bombarded with messages from every form of media, designed to put them in a constant state of arousal.

"What do guys generally want to know about?" I ask.

All at once about twenty-five people yell, "Sex!"

"Right. But what about sex?"

I get a bunch of answers: adequacy, size, duration, where to get some. They're all correct.

"With guys, it's all about their adequacy. Guys want to know if they're normal, if they're doing it right. What about women? What do they want to know?"

"Sex!" a couple guys call out.

"Not quite," I say.

"Relationships," a young woman in front says.

"Yes," I say. "But women are vastly more complex creatures, and so not only do they want to know about relationships, they want to know specifics about men. How do they work? How could he be like that? How come he doesn't behave the way they said he would in the magazine I read? Why is my boyfriend so into lesbians? Why does he want a threesome?"

The subject matter is irresistible. Within minutes, hands are up. This is my favorite part of any talk. In this nonjudgmental atmosphere, the students are open, graphically so. One girl asks why women can't talk about masturbation. I let her tell her story and express her views for a few moments before asking, "Who says women can't talk about it?"

"What do you mean?" she asks, perplexed.

"You're talking about it in front of seven hundred and fifty people," I say.

A mix of laughter, applause, and other sex-related questions follows, giving me a chance to clear up a few myths and mysteries about men and women when it comes to sex. Men are easy to please, I tell them: Most guys are happy if a girl's just there with him. Period. If she's having sex with him, even better. He's ecstatic. Don't worry. He's fine.

"Men are like a machine with a single wheel," I say. "We're not dumb. We're not bad. We're just kind of lame."

"By comparison, women are Rubik's Cubes. They're complicated, hard to figure out, each one unique and different. Yet the popular media tells women they are supposed to function like seventeen-year-old guys. They're supposed to be as into sex as their male counterparts and experience sex in precisely the same way. They feel inadequate when they don't measure up to this male version of sexuality. When they don't respond the way *Cosmo* says they should, they feel flawed and inhibited from expressing their feelings about it."

I follow that with an example.

"Where's the guy who told me he's dumping his girlfriend because she can't have an orgasm?" I ask, referring to a young man who had asked a question earlier.

I scan the faces as best I can, hoping he raises his hand or shouts out. He does. He's a thick-looking guy, built like a rugby player, with short hair and a blue Lacoste shirt and jeans. After explaining that I believe in teaching and learning from our experiences, he allows me to serve him up as a guinea pig.

"What do you think is missing from the equation with you and your girlfriend?" I ask. "What do you think women want in order to have a satisfying sexual experience?"

He thinks for a moment.

"Tommy Lee?" he says.

"No. Try again."

"A Mercedes," he jokes.

"He's getting laughs, and that's good," I say. "But in all seriousness, women want a connected experience. They want meaning. They want feelings."

This is an important point. I sidetrack a bit, though, explaining that so much of what I do at the hospital concerns patients who, due to early life traumas, aren't able to have genuine relationships or connected experiences. Why should this concern a bunch of Ivy League students? Because, like everyone else their age, they have been raised in a pop culture that puts little stock in genuine relationships or connected experiences. It is all about feeling good, getting pumped, going nuts . . . chasing the big *wahoo* moment.

They may think they're immune, but I wouldn't bet on it. I ask them to take a look at their social encounters on campus. I think this is probably the most important portion of my whole talk, as everybody in the audience can relate. According to everything I know, campus social relationships break down into three main groups: a) hooking up, b) joined at the hip, and c) friends with benefits.

I see people agreeing with me.

"In youth culture today, hooking up is the primary means of making contact," I say. "Guys tell me they get loaded so they can get the job done more effectively. The women tell me they get loaded to tolerate the situation because they have to contend with loaded guys hitting on them.

" 'Friends with benefits' is one of the other two unhappy choices for women," I go on. "The other is 'joined at the hip.' Both always end in disaster. Who is benefiting in these rapidly developing relationships? The sex isn't good. The bonds aren't strong. The drama in the relationship is the arousing drug.

"I was once with a group of twelve-to-fourteen-year-olds who insisted that you needed three hookups—which to them usually included oral sex—before you could consider yourself boyfriend and girlfriend."

Half the audience groans. The other half nods in recognition.

"I had an interesting experience at the last high school I spoke at," I say. "A sixteen-year-old girl came up to me after a similar discussion about hooking up and said she got loaded because she was unable to tolerate all the sloppy drunk guys trying to hook up with her. 'I hate those drunk guys,' she said. I asked what she would prefer from men. She said, 'Well, it would be nice if someone would just spend some time talking to me.' Let's say she enjoyed the conversation, I asked; would she want to do it again with him? 'Sure,' she said. At that point, I said, 'Do you understand you're describing a date?'"

Most of the women listening show their approval; the majority of the guys hem and haw, uncertain how to react. The way things stand, the guys have a good deal going—at least in the short term. In the long run, though, no one benefits. None of the relationships are real, deep, or lasting. These kids might find plenty of immediate gratification, but they're never going to get the satisfaction of a genuine relationship from these shallow hookups.

"I see heads nodding out there," I say. "It's like being a drug addict. You always need more, more, more. You're always feeling out of control."

By the end, I have covered an enormous amount of material. The average mom and dad would be shocked to hear their straight-A offspring talking about X, orgasms, threesomes, and hooking up for a night, but I drive home a message that would comfort Grandma and Grandpa: Life isn't all about fun and sex. It can be even better. Slow down. Listen to your inner voice when it comes to right and wrong. Think for yourself. Be more human.

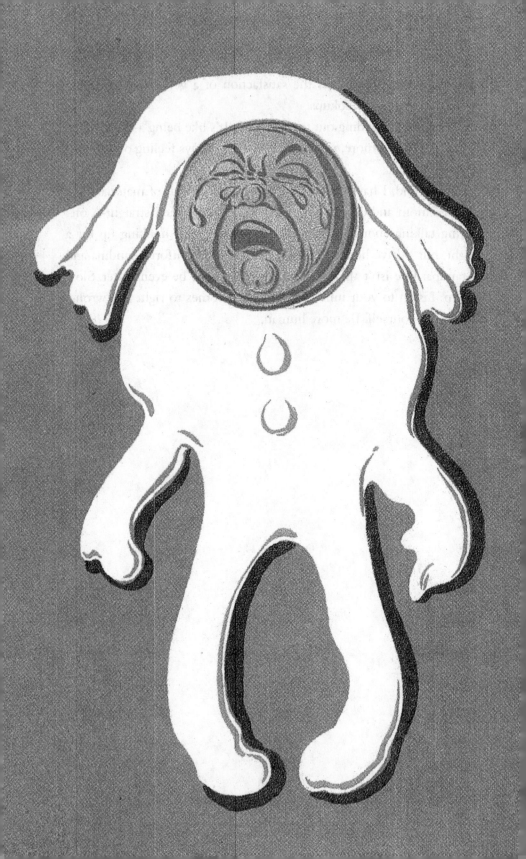

Eleven

WHEN I GET off the airplane I feel half dead, and wonder how I'm going to get up for work the next day. But come sunrise I'm back in the routine, starting out the morning at my private practice. I have one message from a woman asking if she can substitute generic hypertension pills for those I originally prescribed, and another saying that Beverly Norton called, wanting me to know that her husband, Richard, had a pretty good day yesterday. The last message is from Tina Markow, an eighty-one-year-old woman recovering from shingles but suffering from the depression that commonly follows. She wants me to call.

I dial the number and get her daughter. All of a sudden it's good-bye jet lag, hello everyone else's problems. After reminding me that she's an occupational therapist, the daughter complains that her mother doesn't have any energy. Listening to her dire description of her mother's various problems, I get a good idea of what is really going on. I ask a number of questions just to make sure.

By the end of the session, I'm pretty confident about what's really happening here: The daughter is having a difficult time dealing with her mother's failing health. No surprise: It *is* hard, mentally, physically, and emotionally, to watch your parents in decline. The demands are enormous. The responsibility is huge. And when the relationship between parent and child is close, as I gather theirs is, things only get more difficult.

I try to help her understand the real reasons for her mother's lack of energy: She's past eighty, has congestive heart failure, and was nearly done in by a painful, debilitating bout of shingles. She's recovered nicely. But she's old and frail, and she will never be the same. That's reality.

Absorbing that kind of reality is something many find hard to do. As a culture, we're woefully disconnected from the biological reality of our lives. We are born, and then, at some point we can't predict, we die. Like Dr. Finley always reminds me, "There's never a perfect time to be born, to die, or to have a child." We are biological organisms that operate for a finite amount of time. Those are the facts of the human condition, and we don't have any control over them. The one thing we can do is exert some control over what we do with our lives between birth and death.

That's the enormous lesson I try to communicate to patients. A person who's addicted to drugs or alcohol needs to know that all is not lost. They aren't helpless, but they are powerless over their disease.

I'm called to Linsey's room soon after I arrive at the unit.

Alexi is already in her room, hovering nearby. Linsey is curled up in a fetal position on the bed, her knees pulled tightly to her chest, her torso twisted; she claws at the sheets so feverishly I'm surprised they aren't ripped into shreds. Alexi and I get on either side of the bed and try to get her attention, but Linsey is out of control, and she doesn't respond to our efforts. She's facedown, crying into the pillow. I shake her, trying to snap her out of the dissociative state she seems to be in.

She turns over.

"Breathe!" I tell her.

I see panic in her eyes.

"I—I—I don't know what's happening to me," she gasps between sobs.

Linsey appears to be depersonalizing, a strange scary feeling where people feel as though they have ceased to exist. They sometimes describe feeling as though the world is unreal, or as if they're watching it on a movie screen. Dr. Finley arrives, surveys the situation, and confirms my impression. Leaving Linsey in Alexi's capable hands, we step into the hall, where he shares a little additional information about her from an interview he did the other day, as well as notes from the counselors that led her groups.

"She has a borderline history, with a lot of trauma and PTSD, either one of which is like a ticking time bomb when a patient is going through detox," he says.

"Of course," I say. The biological effects of withdrawal tend to amplify this sort of patient's tendency to shift rapidly between intense emotional states. What's happened is that Linsey has frozen in the midst of overwhelming feelings. That is typical. Sometimes that involves dissociation, a biological response that's an evolutionary remnant of the risky strategy of feigning death. That sounds like Linsey.

We go back into her room, where Alexi is trying to soothe the patient, without much success.

"I want to wake up," Linsey cries. "Why can't I wake up?"

Occasionally patients are bad enough that we might transfer them to the hospital's acute psychiatric wing, but we can handle Linsey's condition on our unit. She's not dangerous to herself or others. What she requires is patience and special handling, which Alexi does with textbook calm.

"You're in a safe place," Alexi says, rubbing Linsey's back.

Finley and I debate whether to give her any medication. He says no; he's concerned that she needs to learn how to handle her anxiety. I wonder if she might be too overwhelmed to handle anything right now. I suggest giving her medication to suppress the symptoms contributed by withdrawal. "None of the pharmacotherapy I suggest is meant to gratify," I emphasize.

Linsey eventually goes to sleep. Later, she can't remember anything specific about the episode, though she does complain of feeling spaced out and scared.

"I feel so small," she says in a soft, weepy voice. "I don't know if I can stand any more of this."

"Come to the staff when you feel like that. You've got to trust us. Let them in. Learn to connect with them."

I don't know how much she can comprehend. Not a lot, I'm sure. Nonetheless, I explain that her fragile internal self had been overcome by runaway biology and stress. She's curious about why it happened. I can't say. But I notice a copy of Hemingway's *For Whom the Bell Tolls* on her nightstand, and that may be a clue: provocative, emotional material, of the kind found in a good, challenging novel, can precipitate such episodes.

"You might have felt as if you passed through a dream," I say.

"A nightmare is more like it," she says. "I felt myself slipping away into . . . into like what I said before, nothingness."

Her description is a good one. It makes sense. Growing up, she never received the emotional nourishment needed to build a competent self. To her, "normal" meant feeling helpless, empty, and powerless. On even her best days, she wasn't present in her own life. At her worst, as she had just experienced, she ceased to exist. She was dead, but conscious of it. How frightening is that?

"Scary stuff," I say.

"I want my mom," she sniffles.

"But earlier you told me you didn't want her involved in your treatment. You said she makes things worse."

"I never really even *had* her," says Linsey.

I encourage her to stay with that realization. If I'm correct, Linsey feels terribly alone, even as she's aching for a relationship she never had. She wants connections, and she will have to work at developing them. We are going to help her. Though weak and confused, she nods at my explanation. I can't tell what she means, if she even understands. She probably doesn't. But at least it's a start.

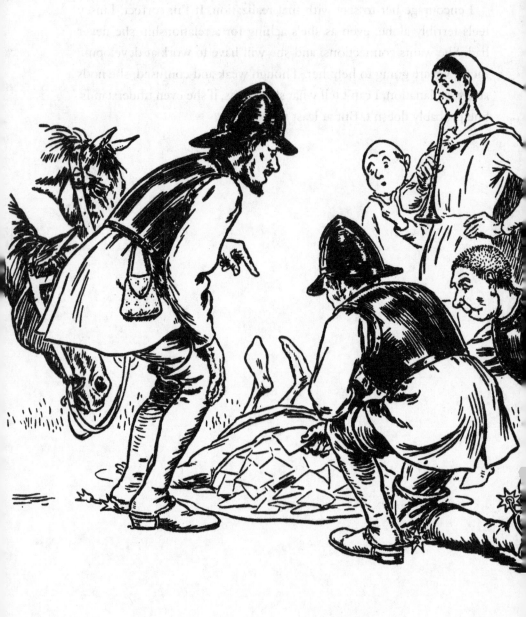

Twelve

ON HER WAY to have lunch, Amber suffers the first in a series of flashbacks. The second episode occurs later that afternoon. Two weeks of treatment are taking a toll. Amber's weight has dropped slightly, and she looks even more fragile than when she came in. The flashbacks are the worst thus far. These explicit visual memories of her abuse intrude upon her consciousness frequently, and without warning. They are probably what motivated her to use in the first place, long before she became addicted.

After dealing with the latest attack, Alexi stomps into the nursing station, where I am filling out paperwork. "She's possessed," she declares.

No, she is traumatized. "Those are the actual symptoms replaying themselves," I say. "Can you imagine? They're causing panic and anxiety at a time when her brain is already twitching from the effects of withdrawal."

Getting through addiction is a roller coaster through hell, and this girl has the front seat on the lead car. It will be weeks before the burning and trembling sensations she complains about start to dissipate. It'll be even longer, many months, before she sleeps soundly.

But that's only one of the afternoon's amusements. A few minutes earlier we took in a new admission. Before I check him out, I ask Alexi for her opinion of him. She opens a can of soda, then glances across the ceiling, as if she's following the flight of an invisible airplane as it arcs across the sky and then crashes into the distance. "He gave off bad vibes," she says.

I feel them, too, as soon as I meet him. Matty's a big, strapping, muscular guy in a Metallica T-shirt, jeans, and work boots. He is twenty-eight, and his résumé includes a two-year history of GHB, a synthetic liquid downer with properties similar to Valium, that's become popular with clubgoers and athletes. I have seen a lot of GHB and speed use in major league ballplayers. Just a Dixie-cup-sized dose can result in the same type of intoxication as a six-pack of beer.

Matty fills the room, even though he's just sitting on a chair. He sits as if posing for a photographer. I sense he is enamored of his own muscular physique. He likes himself. I understand what Alexi meant by "bad vibes." I can envision him cruising the unit as if it were a pickup joint. It won't be long before this guy is acting out in a big way.

"Ever used anabolic steroids?" I ask.

"I've dabbled," he says.

"By any chance, are you a pro ballplayer?"

He laughs. "No, I work in aerospace."

Matty has come for treatment after going through some pretty significant upheavals in his life. A week earlier he had spent an entire day hammering boards over his windows, convinced that his boss, his mother, and his girlfriend had him under surveillance. Then, just the other night, he lost control at a bar and got into a fight. The cops taking him away found a trace amount of speed in his pocket.

"How much GHB have you been doing?" I ask.

"Three capfuls a day, give or take," he says.

Acting as if my questions are a distraction, he starts checking out his right bicep. He flexes and moves his arm in different positions. He seems mesmerized. I sense his resistance, his cockiness, his disregard for anything other than his own gratification. His type is oblivious to the pain he causes in other people.

"Marijuana?"

"A little in high school," he says. "It made me paranoid." This from a guy who was boarding up his windows just a few days earlier because he thought surveillance planes were spying on him.

"Cocaine?" I ask, scrolling through a routine drug history.

"I had a run-in about four years ago for a summer."

"Speed?"

"Occasionally."

"How often?"

"I don't know. Maybe two or three times a week. But I started smoking it lately, so maybe I've been doing a little more."

He's not bashful about answering questions, that's for sure. He sits openly, true to character, his body language telling me to ask him anything. He started doing speed two years earlier. In the beginning it was a tool that helped him maintain his social life and work. Then the addiction kicked in. (I see a lot of students doing the same thing to help them through crazy study hours. They don't understand that methamphetamine, like X, is one of those drugs that damages the brain. It causes mood problems and impairs memory. So much for academic performance.)

"You need to be willing to consider that these thoughts and problems you have had have been caused by the drugs you've been using. It's typical of speed. Sometimes using only two or three times a week causes a slow, intense delusional preoccupation, and it's almost always with family, co-workers, friends, and neighbors. You think they're all talking about you."

"I know it sounds crazy, but you need to hear this story," he says. "We live by the airport. My girlfriend knows this guy who works in air traffic control, and one day he shows up at our house. He used to work for the FBI—"

Matty ended up thinking the entire L.A. bureau had him under watch. This is a pretty typical delusion among speed addicts. They all start with some innocent observation, around which they construct elaborate fantasies. The creativity and the detail are always astounding. It's like John Nash, the character Russell Crowe played in the film *A Beautiful Mind*. The stories are easy to believe—to a point. I don't think the U.S. government is too concerned about Matty, but he thought otherwise.

"I bet these experiences are taking a toll on your relationship with your mom and your girlfriend," I say.

"Well, that's why I'm here. I had to promise them I'd get help."

"Good, that's a good move," I say. "I bet you've been really uncomfortable. You're going to start to feel better with some more time off the drugs."

"So I hang out here a while," he says, nodding. "Cool. Just like my lawyer said."

"There's a lot of other personal work we'll want you to do."

"Whatever," he says with a shrug. "This place doesn't seem too bad. And some of the patients are kind of hot." When I don't react, he adds, "Just kidding."

Except I know he's serious. Over the next couple days, he bothers a number of women in the unit, both patients and staff, with strongly sexual, highly inappropriate remarks. Alexi issues a stern warning: Either tone it down or leave. Of course, that can only have so much effect; after all, he is out of control.

As dislikable as the situation is, we can't forget that Matty is sick. His harassment is a symptom of the disease that has brought him here. Sexuality is another drug for many addicts, another means of activating the brain's arousal apparatus to escape or manage unpleasant feel-ings. Sex makes Matty feel good. It's like a pill. Women for him are merely sources of gratification; there isn't much difference to him between compulsive drug use and compulsive sex.

Still, his behavior disturbs people. After another complaint from a nurse, one of many, I have to talk to him. As I head toward his room, I think how convenient and efficient it would be to simply kick him out. Good-bye; no more complaints. I can't, though. He hasn't vio-lated any rules. He has just been obnoxious. So when I find Matty reading an old *Sports Illustrated* and greeting me as if I were a friend picking him up on the way to happy hour at the corner bar, it occurs to me to try to connect with him, in the hope of getting him to start following directions.

"Have you had any long relationships?" I ask.

"Yeah, after I left college," he says. "There was this great girl who lived across the hall from me. She was the greatest. I really loved her. We hung out together. She was always around if I needed her. We'd have sex pretty often, and there were no strings attached. What do they call that now?"

"Friends with benefits," I say.

"Yeah. Perfect description." He laughs.

"Have you ever had a sexually transmitted disease?"

He brushes some of his black hair to the side. "About a year or so after college, I had warts. The doctor gave me something. My friend, she got upset when she got them, too. But no big deal, you know? We were friends. She understood."

"There were other women, too, right?"

"I had other friends, sure. I slept with some of them."

"How long were you with this girl?"

"Around a year, I guess. Eventually she started taking things seri-ously. Even though I was always honest with her, she seemed to want a relationship."

"After being together a year, what did you think you had?"

"A friendship. An understanding. I was always up front about that. But then she developed feelings for me, and that wasn't what we'd agreed on. Then I had another girlfriend who did that, too. She was this hot dancer. One day she just flipped out. We had to break that off."

I can imagine that nightmare. The stripper. Drugs. Arguments about commitment.

"Dr. Pinsky—just so you know, my girlfriend now is the greatest."

"How so?"

"She doesn't pressure me or anything. She lets me do what I want."

"Did she want you to come in for treatment?"

"Oh, yeah. She was real supportive. She and my mom have been talking."

"Does she talk to your father, too?"

"My dad? Who knows where *that* asshole is?"

"Will we see your girlfriend in family groups here?"

"Family groups? I don't know. But she'll bring me stuff all the time. Anytime I want something."

Perfect. He has a servant, a puppy dog at his disposal. I don't know this woman, but I'll bet she learned that caretaker role early, perhaps growing up with an alcoholic father. Other than the relationship she's forged with his mother, she's not much different from the stripper who came before her. She's just dancing better.

I've heard this story before, so I know the dynamics of his personal life. His girlfriend tolerates him in order to maintain the status quo. She doesn't want to lose him. She has her own issues. But there's no real relationship, no discussion of feelings, needs, or love. Matty would find that too much of a hassle.

I wonder if he has any idea.

"How does she deal with all of your bullshit?"

"You know what? She was great until I got picked up after the fight."

★ ★ ★

Later, I realize I'm worked up about Matty. It's a delayed reaction. Talking to him put me into a blue funk. He's in such deep denial that I can't conceive of him getting anything positive from treatment. I hate to say that, but it's true. It makes me feel I'm wasting as much time as the patient. My depression is compounded when I see Matty on the patio, talking and smoking with Amber. Then he moves on to another table and more women. It's just a matter of time until he attempts to prey upon one of them.

Finley, as is his way, catches me at my worst and scoops me up like a flapping fish. I unload. I'm terribly conflicted. Yes, I am supposed to be treating Matty, but I have a serious aversion toward the guy. He uses women to gratify himself, and he does it without any regard for the consequences. He doesn't appear to have any conscience about his behavior. Okay, out of pure frustration, I try to look at things another way. *Maybe I'm jealous, I think. Maybe I wish a part of me could act on every primitive urge I felt.*

"Drew, you couldn't be less of a caveman," Finley laughs. "You don't like this guy. End of story."

"Yeah, you're right," I say. "As I think about it, I thought, I might be reacting most strongly to what Matty represents. He's a little older, but he epitomizes the whole hooking-up culture that's screwing kids up all over. I was just talking about that with those students at Princeton."

"What's wrong with our culture?" Finley asks. "Where have we gone?"

"This is what depresses me," I say. "Because I think we created it. I don't know if we aren't guilty. We opened the door in the 1970s. We celebrated sex, drugs, and rock and roll. We fantasized about what the freedom rock gods and movies stars had. That was me back in 1978. The Amherst student newspaper described the typical male student as athletic, intelligent, a beer in one hand, the other hand searching for a breast to grab onto. Get high, get laid. That was the rallying cry every weekend."

"It was innocent."

"It was misinformed. It's not healthy. And instead of learning from our mistakes, we made the music faster and louder, and the drugs stronger and cheaper."

"Go home, Drew," Finley says. "Put on an easy-listening station. Stop at all the red lights. Keep the world righteous."

"Go ahead, make fun. I don't care," I say.

It's nice to know I can leave the craziness and go home where the TV is on, the kids are doing homework, my wife has got things under control, and everything is disorderly, hectic, and enjoyably normal. It is a short drive home from the unit. When I walk in, Susan is preparing dinner; the kids are doing their homework, and arguing about what they're going to watch on television later.

I know this Normal Rockwell sort of family scene is fragile and precious. In 1995, we were vacationing as a family in Las Vegas when it was nearly torn apart. The children were horsing around in the hotel room when Douglas jumped off the bed and struck his head squarely on the floor. He lay motionless on the ground while the rest of us freaked out, me included. He began coming around by the time the paramedics arrived and rushed him to the hospital. There doctors found a cyst in his cerebellum, which had moved in the fall and momentarily knocked out his brain stem function.

With Douglas in the hospital and seriously ill, we consulted with specialists and plotted a course of treatment. A few days later we transported Douglas to Los Angeles, where surgeons at Children's Hospital put a window in the cyst, allowing the cerebrospinal fluid to flow freely from the cyst. Douglas has been fine ever since.

My recovery has taken much longer. The emergency opened that old Pandora's box of fears about the dangers I'm convinced are always out there waiting to happen to me. The repercussions drove everyone crazy. I was like my mother had been with me. My mother wouldn't let me have sleepovers. She practically broke into tears as I pedaled my bike around the block. Now I started acting the same way; I didn't want the kids riding their bikes anywhere, lest something happen to them. I never got as bad as my mother, but Susan still forced me to spend a little time in therapy.

And now? Nobody's perfect, including me. I still go from *all's well* to *the end is near* faster than anyone west of Woody Allen. Doesn't matter that I spend half my day instructing patients to have faith that things will work out, I still expect to walk around the corner and be confronted by the worst. Consider tonight. Dinner is great, the conversation boisterous, and when the kids go to bed I marvel at how they can lay their heads down and fall asleep instantaneously. I run through a quick catalog of my fears. Will one of us get into a car accident? What about the flu? Then I turn my attention to the unit. Matty's driving me crazy, but I would like to help him. What about Amber? She's really going through a tough time. And Linsey? Did I do a good job? Am I doing all I can for these people? What about tomorrow? Admittedly, this is a none-too-healthy burden to shoulder on a daily basis. I'm just lucky that my fears of crisis are usually proved wrong.

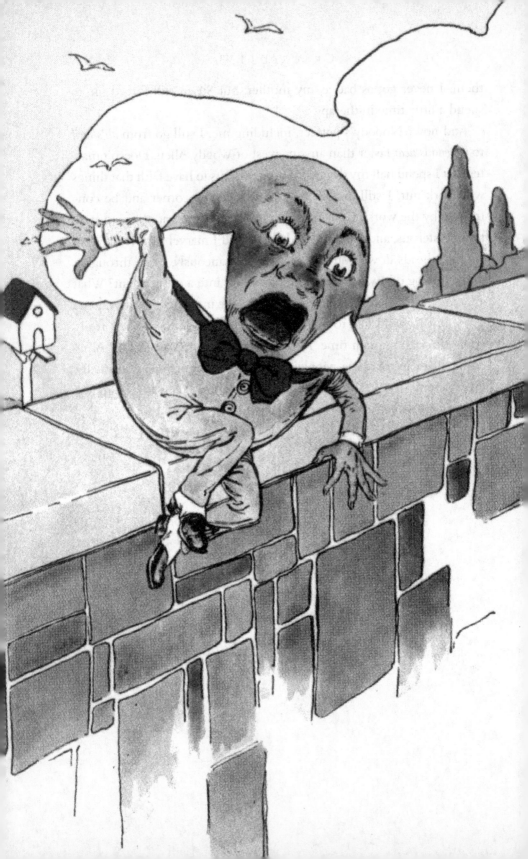

Thirteen

"DID YOU KNOW Katherine gave me a good-bye hug?" I say, in a tone meant to convey surprise. Seated in the conference room with the unit's treatment team, I'm sharing the unexpected gesture from the cell-phone fiend with my long-suffering colleagues. Almost everyone on the team—Finley, Alexi, the unit's two chemical dependency counselors, the family program rep, the nutritionist, and our utilization and review nurse—smiles in surprise at the story.

"The wicked witch of the east?" says Gail, a counselor in her midfifties who has years of sobriety under her belt.

The treatment team meets weekly to update each patient's progress. We also use the time to let off steam. Everything said in the room stays there.

"Her husband came out to take her to Sober Living back east," I say.

"Were they flying commercial?" asks Debra, the other counselor, grinning. "Or did he bring her broom?"

"He's in therapy, too. And the fact that she leaves with a positive attitude about treatment is an important prognostic sign," Finley says. "Drew, did you check in on Maria?"

Maria is a returning heroin addict. Admitted a week earlier, she's going through the motions just as she's done numerous times before.

"Yes," I say. "She can't sleep."

"She wants meds all the time," interjects Alexi.

"Has anyone gotten a whiff of her?" says Gail, the utilization nurse. "Pee-yew."

"I don't care what she says, she's sleeping," says Debra. "She's a liar. Her whole life is a lie."

"Insurance?" asks Finley.

"Covered," says Gail.

"What about Amber?" asks Finley, opening a new chart.

"I don't know," says Alexi. "She has some good moments, but she's having flashbacks. And she's still at the window."

"Has anyone met her husband?" says Pat. "That guy comes in here and gets her and everyone else worked up."

"Still?" I ask.

"Shoot him," says Alexi.

"Drew, he talks about you like you're best friends," says Pat.

"With friends like that . . ." I respond. "She's far enough in her withdrawal that she should be settling down."

"She's not."

"Let's try reducing her meds. I'll reduce the dose, but make the intervals more frequent."

"I'd like add something," says Debbie, the nutritionist. "She has an eating disorder. She's eating about thirty percent of her tray, and she's put on six pounds since admission."

"Six pounds?" I say. "That doesn't sound right." I glance through her med sheet to see if any of her medications could be causing fluid retention. "I'm concerned. If she keeps gaining weight, she may start to preoccupy about it and trigger purging."

"Aside from her husband, what's the family situation?" asks Finley.

"Supposedly she contacted her mother," Alexi says. "But I don't know if there's going to be any involvement."

"She's going to groups," says Gail. "She's labile and has trouble tracking, but she attends. She's started to participate."

"Obstacles to recovery?" Finley asks, getting to the bottom of his checklist.

"That husband of hers," Alexi says.

"Poor family support," Pat adds.

"Limited financial resources," Gail says.

The negatives pile up, but I don't want to hear them.

"If we can just get her adequately enrolled and connected," I say. "I don't know why, but I see something in her."

"I like her, too," Alexi says. "As sick as she is, there's something about her that's likable."

"Agreed," Pat says.

Alexi looks at me. "But—"

Finley closes Amber's chart and selects the next one in the pile. Everyone in the room moves on, except for me. I continue to think about Amber, wondering what it's going to take for her to get it. I review everything I know about her, and ask myself if I'm doing everything I can to help.

Later I receive a call that disturbs me, both as a parent and as a doctor, because I've been consulted on situations just like it more times than I care to remember. I hear the concern in the man's voice. It's a tone I've heard countless times from other parents.

"It's my son, Barry," he says. "He's eighteen."

"What's wrong?" I ask.

"Somebody slipped him something. Or gave him something."

"What's happening right now?"

"He's psychotic. He's locked in the bathroom. He thinks everyone is trying to kill him. His muscles are rigid. He goes in and out of it."

"Do you have any idea what he took?"

"No."

"Has he been depressed or had any other psychiatric symptoms lately?"

I hear a click on the phone line. His wife has picked up an extension.

"He's had a couple panic attacks," she says. "From the stress of school."

I don't buy that.

"Do you know if he does any drugs? Is he into the club scene or that sort of thing?"

"Yes, he's smoked pot," says his mother. "What kid these days doesn't? But he doesn't do it that often. And he seems to be fine with it. As far as the clubs, sure, he's very social and has lots of friends. Barry's a great kid. He's a B-plus student at the University of Colorado."

What does one thing have to do with another? Nothing. I get scared thinking of how many parents I speak to who only know their children by their SAT scores.

"He's also locked in your bathroom, lying on the floor and scared that you want to kill him."

His father clears his throat.

"Barry's younger brother said that Barry was supposed to be taking Ecstasy. He thought someone must've given him something else."

"Maybe, but I don't think so," I say. "From your description, it sounds like something I've seen before from Ecstasy. Severe psychotic reactions can be precipitated by this drug. In addition, there can be something called the posthallucinogenic perceptual disorder, where people can feel like they're locked into the effects of the drug, unable to escape. At some point they then start to feel panicky, then paranoid, and eventually their moods hit the skids. Often the mood problems persist."

"Oh my God," says his mother.

"I don't want to overwhelm you with information," I continue, "but I bet you there's a marijuana problem here as well."

"So what do we do?" asks his father.

"I'd bring him here to the hospital immediately," I say.

The biggest problem with Ecstasy is the lack of information surrounding the drug and its side effects. Even first-time users who have a great experience usually report intense depression the next day. They get a great big high, and then an equally significant low. They go from one extreme to the other. Often the depression lingers.

If you've seen anyone the day after using X, you know why they're referred to as E-tards. They're listless, moody, scattered. They're being one hundred percent accurate when they say they're burned out. After one large hit or about twenty regular doses, users suffer mood changes. Barry's reaction was atypical, but I have seen people present like this, suddenly psychotic, often with muscle stiffness, like Parkinsonism. The more common syndrome is a social person who gradually isolates, then develops panic and agoraphobia, followed by a quick and persistent plummet of mood.

Young people who hear me speak about the realities of X often get angry. They squirm at the sight of a CAT scan showing the lesions just a couple of exposures leave on the brain. They ask, "Why hasn't anyone told us this before?"

Then, because at eighteen or twenty years old you think you're impervious to everything, someone will invariably ask how many times they can use X before suffering side effects. We don't know for sure, but in my experience the potentially lifelong effects usually start after fifteen to twenty times. But there's no definitive answer. Anyone doing X is playing Russian roulette. They're not only tempting fate, they're fooling with bad science.

By chance, a few hours later, we admit a good example of this. Chloe is eighteen years old. She has black hair with purple highlights, a couple of tattoos on her arms, and a piercing under her lower lip. Despite the adornments, she appears younger and more innocent than I imagine she really is.

I rarely see people her age who aren't scared about what's happening to them, though amazingly they manage to avoid their fears until they come to treatment and start getting better. Then every hangnail is a crisis. Chloe's no exception. Three days earlier, she explains, she took GHB. She hasn't come down yet. She still feels racy. She has prickly sensations up and down her arms and legs. She can't sleep. I also notice that she's mildly paranoid, and her speech is somewhat garbled. She has trouble maintaining a linear thought. She moves constantly. Even sitting still, her leg is jumping up and down.

"How'd you get going on GHB?" I ask; it's unusual to see someone using that drug alone.

"I really wasn't doing it that often," she says. "Maybe three or four times a week. I did it at night to get myself in a better mood before going out."

That figures. GHB is a party drug. It's like having a few beers before hitting the scene. But it sneaks up slowly on users. They start craving the subtle euphoria.

"Were you also doing X?" I ask.

"A few times," she says. "Last year in high school."

"Once? Three times? More? How many times did you use it?"

"I don't know. Four or five times over the past couple years."

"Could it be more than four or five times?" I ask, knowing it's more likely at least ten to fifteen.

"I don't know, " she says. "Maybe. I can't remember."

"How was it the first time you took it?"

"Great. I had a great time."

"How'd you feel the next day?"

"Depressed."

"Let me give you some facts," I say, looking directly into her eyes She makes strong contact in return—a good sign. "With X, that depression can be permanent. Sometimes it can be fifteen hits or one big one. You never know. It leaves you with a groggy, sluggish, depressed feeling that never goes away. You might be on the verge."

I can see her fear surface in her eyes as she fights back tears. I take her hand and give it a comforting squeeze.

Chloe follows the pattern of a number of young GHB users. Over the next two days, she comes back to earth. She doesn't have much detox experience to endure, though she receives a small amount of medication to deal with the paranoia, agitation, and hyperexcitability. Then she wakes up two days later feeling so much better that she wants to leave. In one of our last talks, she resists the idea that GHB is addictive.

"I've never been addicted to anything," she argues.

"I think you should go to meetings," I say.

"But it's not a problem," she says.

Actually, most GHB users don't crave the drug after a few weeks off it, and indeed often grow afraid of it. But the residual effects can linger for months, in the form of crankiness, irritability, and generally manic behavior. Inevitably they start using again, and that itself can open them up to treatment. Looking at her bag all packed, I put Chloe in this category.

"How about your parents?" I ask.

"They're divorced," she says.

"Do either of them have any problems with drugs or alcohol?"

"My mom likes to smoke a little pot now and then. She likes it for sex. My dad's an alcoholic."

She's dealing with that same thing. She just doesn't know it. She hasn't gotten her wake-up call yet. There's not much I can do. She's up and out of here, though before she leaves, I warn her that there will likely come a time when she'll need to face facts. I don't want her to be blind to them.

"You may not be ready to look at this now," I say. "But you inherited a biology from your dad that set you up for this. You are an addict.

I know you don't think of yourself that way. I know you don't feel like you have a problem. So you may have to try this on your own. But please, do both of us a favor and remember this conversation, before too much shit rains down on you. It'll save you more problems."

"Thanks, Dr. Drew—uh, Dr. Pinsky."

"Good-bye, Chloe. Good luck."

Not long after that call I remember that I haven't yet seen Barry, the teenage X casualty. If his parents had followed my advice, they would have brought him right here to the hospital. Hadn't he been paralyzed on the bathroom floor? Didn't he believe that his family wanted to kill him. Aren't either of those reasons to seek help?

My guess was that Barry was suffering from more than an allergic reaction. From their description, I'd bet he would spend two or three days cooling off in the locked unit. Once his psychosis had settled down, he would be brought onto our unit, where we would continue to require medication while he went through withdrawal, from marijuana, I suspect. Then we'd get him into groups so he could start learning to make connections that would help him manage the feelings that had originally ignited his addiction back when he first started smoking pot.

They hadn't mentioned a pot addiction, but I bet Barry had smoked pot daily for the past three or four years. When pot starts losing its effect, addicts like Barry try smoking more, or trade up to better pot or hash. When that doesn't work, they head toward stimulants like speed. Barry had probably done X as often as twice a weekend for six months without any problems until that fateful night. After that, the situation was more dire.

His is a common story. Right now one in five chemical dependency admissions is for marijuana addiction. That's twenty percent. This isn't the casual smoker lighting up once a month. Pot addicts generally have a family history of alcoholism, which they swear they will never touch. They smoke pot instead. The majority of them tell the same story of getting started. Their first time was no big deal. The second was okay. The third was magical. They develop an intimate relationship with their pot. They can't imagine life before this wonderfully soothing herb. I will ask a roomful of pot addicts who remembers the first time they smoked, and no one will raise their hand. If I alter the question slightly by asking who remembers the first time they got high, every single hand shoots up. A pot addict can recall the exact day twenty years later.

But at some point this amazing experience loses its power to sway and seduce. The love affair goes stale. The addict is left depressed and irritable by this biological betrayal, and also confused and panicked. Think about it. If you've managed your moods for twenty years by smoking pot and then suddenly it stops working, what do you do? Start smoking more, smoking better—even though all of that actually accelerates the decline into depression, anxiety, and panic.

Most pot addicts try GHB, LSD, Ecstasy, and mushrooms. This is where Barry was at, I am sure. They are chasing that high, that soothing sensation that sheltered them from real feelings. Eventually the typical pot addict graduates to speed. Amphetamines seem to work best when it comes to lifting them from the depression caused by chronic marijuana use, and from there it's all bad news.

I want the latest on Barry, and soon enough curiosity gets the better of me. I call Alexi, who has wisely saved the father's callback number for me. I make the call from my den at home. As the telephone rings, I figure the couple must have taken their son someplace else, which is fine with me. I merely want to follow up, find out if Barry is doing better, and answer any questions they might have. Treatment can be as confusing as any medical procedure.

The father answers; he sounds as if I caught him a little off guard, but his tone is friendly and open. He thanks me for checking in, even cracks a joke about how these days you can wait six hours or more in an emergency room for a doctor to see you and yet here I am actually calling a patient at home.

That's my cue. Much to my surprise, I remind him, his son never became a patient. "What happened?" I ask.

"He improved some and we took him to the emergency room," he says. "They gave him a shot—"

"They probably sedated the hell out of him," I interrupt.

"But he seemed pretty good," the father continues. "We sent him back up to school yesterday."

"Oh. Okay."

"We really appreciated the way you talked to us when I called. It helped us get a handle on Barry's situation. Then we talked about it at a family meeting. I agree with his brother, who said someone probably slipped Barry something he didn't expect. As for Ecstasy, we explained the facts to him just as you described them to us. We told him that that drug is a time bomb."

"Good," I say.

"Just to be safe, I said, 'Son, you have to be careful nowadays. You don't know what you're getting with these designer drugs. You can't tell. There's no regulation. If you have to do something, stick to your bong.' " He pauses. "Dr. Pinsky, I grew up in the seventies. Things were different then. Safer. Don't you agree?"

No, I don't. I couldn't disagree more. The father's attitude is so disturbing I don't have a response. Not a polite response, anyway. I could read him the riot act. They're convinced they have a handle on the situation, when in reality they're in such denial that their lack of response could end up leading to much more serious problems for their son. Barry might have already suffered brain injury as a result of his drug use. And he could be on the verge of a bigger break.

I end the call politely, wishing him good luck, and then I spend the rest of the night stewing in a quiet rage and disgust.

But the truth is, I have more trouble getting through to parents than their children. A speaking engagement I did at a private L.A. high school is typical. Midway through the presentation, a group of parents took exception to me for suggesting that their children drank, smoked pot, and took X. These parents wanted information, but they thought it was merely preventive. All I could think was, *Wait a minute, here are the facts: Forty percent of high schoolers drink regularly; over fifty percent are using illicit drugs, and one in ten twelfth graders has used Ecstasy. If some of those aren't your kids, whose are they?*

I understood their reaction. The world is a frightening place, and parents don't want to think of their kids experimenting with sex and drugs. But they do, and it's negligent and irresponsible to deny it. As I told those angry parents, I don't tell anyone what to do. I present information that will help you and your children make good, hopefully healthy choices. You have to talk to your kids. You also have to know what you're talking about. I want people to understand the facts when someone is developing momentum in their use of drugs or alcohol. If that happens, I won't get as many calls from parents asking what to do because their kid is passed out on the bathroom floor.

"Let me give you an example," I told those L.A. parents. And then I told them the cautionary tale of Barry. "This boy could have been anyone's kid . . . "

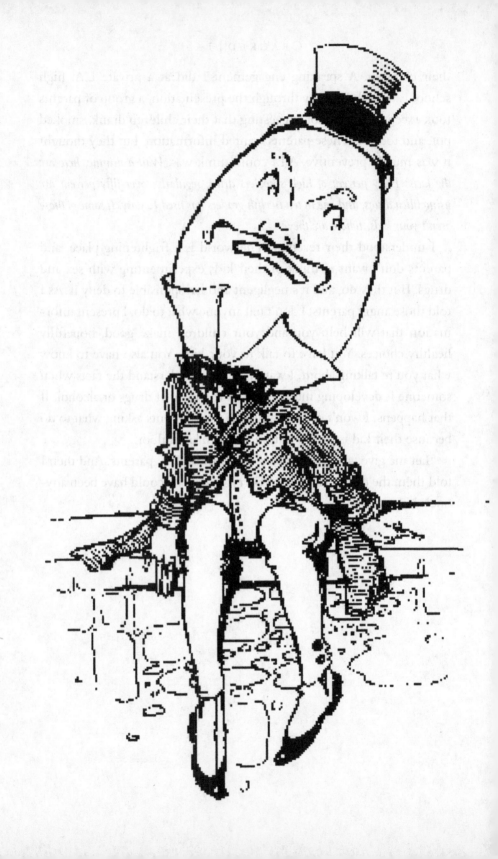

Fourteen

RICHARD NORTON WAS taken to the hospital during the night. His wife, Beverly, left a message with my service in the early morning hours. When I call a few hours later she sounds confused and unsure about the details, though with one sentence she tells me everything I need: The attending cardiologist has recommended no further treatment than necessary to keep him comfortable.

"You know him so well," she says. "We've been with you so long. I wanted to be sure you agreed."

For a moment I fantasize about a transplant operation or other desperate measures, but all are ridiculous in a man of Richard's age. No, all the right things are being done.

"It sounds appropriate," I say. "Please keep me informed. I'll check in, too. Let me know how you're doing."

"Our children are with me," she says. "We're okay."

I spend the short drive to the unit thinking about Richard. He was a warm old man who would come in for an ache or a checkup and leave having made *me* feel better. We spent a lot of time over the years talking about his career selling scrap metal around the world, in places that provided him with great stories made even better by his gift for gab. But the thing I remember most about Richard is his passion for his family. Though he made a nice living, I can still hear him saying that money never bought him the things that gave him pleasure: his children and friends.

"What do you do with your kids?" he once asked me.

"I play with them," I said. "I help with homework. I coach sports. I go to my daughter's skating competitions."

"Good," he said. "We spent a whole lot of time just talking with our children. I think those were the best times of my life."

"I understand," I'd say.

"That's wonderful," he said. "Most people your age don't have a clue."

Neither do I have a clue about the source of the noise I hear when walking into the unit. It turns out to be a soda can bouncing off a wall, which I spot when it rolls out of Room 120. A counselor passing by at the same moment glances at the room and shakes her head, warning me it isn't pretty inside. I trod in warily and remind the patient, Titus Fenton, a medium-built black man with long dreadlocks and thrift-store clothes, that neither his room, the hallway, nor anyplace else in the unit is a trash can. He couldn't care less.

The man looks fifty-two; his chart says he's twenty years younger. That's startling, but not nearly as much as the condition of his room. He has occupied it for not quite three and a half hours, and yet it is layered with clothes, papers, blankets, sheets, and food wrappers. It is a pit. He has also managed to estrange himself from the staff.

"So what's up?" I ask. "Why are you here?"

"I'm strung out," he mutters. "I'm a junkie. My girlfriend made me come."

"Congratulations," I say, already turned off.

"I'll be leaving in two days," he declares. "I'm out of sick days at work. I need the dough. That's my survival, man."

Titus is snappish, rude, scattered, and not aware that his life isn't working for him. All that aside, though, it's hard to like this guy. It's bad chemistry. I'll make sure he's getting the best treatment we can offer. But I'm not going to waste my efforts trying to make a connection. It won't happen, no matter what. When someone like Titus declares that he's history, with this kind of strong conviction, I have no reason to doubt him.

We get a number of patients like Titus. It's part of the disease. They pass in and out, literally and figuratively. They usually aren't nasty to anyone, though; Titus is an exception. Nor do they pose any particular threat, other than stirring up the other patients, as long as they don't bring drugs onto the unit. I am just looking for the smallest shred of desire to get better. He doesn't care about the rules I lay out, because he doesn't intend to deal with them. He has his own game plan. He hasn't figured out that it's a losing proposition.

Titus isn't close to being ready for recovery, but I suspect something else is going on here. He has another agenda aside from recovery. Sometimes we find out later that patients like Titus are using us to hide out from some more immediate threat: the law, process servers, dealers, gambling debts, or their family. Still, as long as Titus doesn't create any major problems on the floor, he can stay. Sometimes all it takes is planting that seed of recovery.

But there are better uses for my time—like my next patient. A single mother of a ten-year-old girl, Hannah is a twenty-eight-year-old from South Pasadena. I suspect I've seen her around, but she says no; then I ask about the Pasadena City College T-shirt she's wearing, and learn that she grew up close to my childhood stomping grounds. Her story also has a familiar ring. She began taking Vicodin after getting a tooth pulled, and it triggered a predisposition that soon became a three-year opiate and benzodiazepine addiction. She tried to kill herself two days ago by overdosing on Ambien, Vicodin, and Xanax. She transferred last night from a nearby emergency room. She's sitting up in bed when I see her, frantically rubbing her arms.

"I feel like I'm climbing out of my skin," she says.

One look and I can see why. Her hands shake involuntarily. Though she doesn't go into the excruciating details, I know she is battling the sensation of a constant, painful sizzle of nerve endings. It's the manifestation of her central nervous system firing up after months of being suppressed by downers. It's as if she's frying from within.

"I'm so depressed. I can't believe what I did," she says in a whimpery voice.

"Tell me what you mean."

"What I did to my daughter when I tried to kill myself."

I take a seat next to her bed. She went to college, she tells me. She wants it known that she's not a tramp. She reads, she says, gesturing to a pile of novels on her nightstand. But living with an addiction, she gradually lost her friends, then her job, and she figured the rest of her life was next. A stint on welfare was followed by a struggle for survival. After deciding she couldn't go on any longer, she decided in a fit of desperation and depression to take her life, and enlisted her daughter's help by having her bring more and more pills from the medicine cabinet, swallowing two at a time until the bottles were empty.

"She kept asking if I was okay," she says. "She thought I was taking too much. But I insisted I was sick, and the doctor told me to do it. I lied." She breaks into tears. "God is going to send me to hell for lying to her like that. Then I told her—her name is Cheryl—to go do her homework and put herself to bed if Mommy fell asleep before her. God, how awful is that? How much did I screw up? How much is my baby going to hate me? I hate myself."

I don't move or say a word. The best thing I can do for her at the moment is to just be there for a few moments so she doesn't feel alone.

"I want you to go to group this afternoon," I say.

She nods.

"My family is coming tonight," she says. "Should my daughter come, too?"

"Yes," I say. "And get her in Alateen."

I can also hear Finley jumping on me to get the girl a therapist. Hopefully there will be insurance resources for such care. No way Hannah can pay herself.

"How long will I be detoxing?"

"Five to seven days."

"Then the shaking will stop?"

"It should."

"There's no more medication, right? I mean, they've given me something. But I can't have anything for the pain, right?"

"That's correct."

As I turn to leave, she stops me with a slight tug on my elbow. She sits up, takes a tissue from the nightstand, wipes her eyes, and then blows her nose.

"Dr. Pinsky," she starts, but then nothing comes out for a few minutes. During the silence, I pull a chair next to the bed and sit down, content to wait. When I think about all the medicine I've practiced over the years, the most useful skill I've managed to develop is patience. A large portion of my job is spent listening to people.

"Dr. Pinsky," she continues. "I'm really, really . . . *really* . . . scared. I don't want to die." She is overcome by tears and needs another moment to regroup before speaking again. "I didn't want to kill myself. But I couldn't take it any longer. I just hate feeling this way. It's ruined my life. I'm so fucked up."

I stand by her bed in silence. I try to express my appreciation of her pain with my expressions. It's hard not to be overcome and invaded by her feelings. My impulse is to rush in and rescue her from her discomfort. I could just medicate it away. But no, my job is just to remain present and reflect my understanding of her distress. This is how she will develop a road map of her emotions, and the capacity to regulate them. And that will reduce her risk of using. I want her to know there are people she can trust not to hurt or exploit her, starting with me.

"We're here to help," I say. "You can trust us. We'll help get you through this."

When I finally return to the nursing station, Alexi hands me a message from my private practice nurse, Angel. It says to call the office. But Alexi delivers the news: My patient Richard has died. For a moment, both of us just look at each other in silence. She knows I'll need a moment to digest the information.

I never thought much about death growing up, and then when I was exposed to it in medical school it was very clinical. Without any kind of personal investment, I couldn't think about it beyond the way I felt about death myself, which has evolved over time. My attitude is matter-of-fact, pragmatic: It's better to be alive than dead, and while you're alive, you should try your best to make the experience rich and meaningful. At the end, you want to be flooded with good memories, with thanks for the people you love and the time you've shared with them. Just as no one ever died wishing they'd spent more time at the office, no one ever died saying, I wish I'd spent more time by myself.

Which makes Richard's story, in the end, a happy one. I hated to hear about his death, but there was something dignified and right about it. He was a great guy, a loving husband, father, grandfather, and friend. Through all those close to him, his life would continue to have meaning. Occasionally I'm asked what, if anything, I know about death beyond the clinical. I usually say there's a lot to learn about death from people who are dying, but in the end they really teach us the value of living, and that's where I place my attention.

I'm not alone. The will to live is instinctual in humans. The will to feel good and exist without pain is just as strong. I see it even in my worst patients. In fact, on my way out I stop by Amber's room. Our eyes connect for a second, and I see terror flash in hers. As soon as I'm in her room, she lets me know she's in pain.

"I need something more to take me down," she says.

It's hard to resist Amber's plea. Something about this young woman is undeniably attractive, not just to me but to a number of us in the unit. She's settled into the routine with some success lately, though she's still regularly overcome by waves of agitation and a periodic desire to bolt. This is clearly one of those moments. "I need to be here," she says. "I feel like I *want to use.* If I go home, I'll use. I will, I swear to God. And it's freaking me out."

I nod, and try to stay with her emotionally. The dynamics of situations like these are intense. Recovery takes months and years of self-help and frequently some psychotherapy, but in this initial phase of treatment, when the goal is getting the patient safely through her unstable medical and psychiatric problems, evaluating her needs, and getting her on track, a single moment can start the turnaround.

I don't think Amber is there yet. She's caught in the struggle of wanting to live and knowing she might die if she makes the wrong choice. As a doctor, I'm trained to help. But sometimes I can't do anything more than be there and offer support. It's a strange situation: She's struggling to find the strength to fight her addiction, and I know that better than she does, but ultimately there's only so much I can do to help. In the end, she has to summon the strength and do it herself.

"Can't you give me something?" she pleads.

"I'm doing everything that's right for you."

And so the day ends, patient and doctor together.

Neither with the answer.

Humpty Dumpty
sat on a Wall
Humpty Dumpty
had a great fall

Fifteen

LINSEY THINKS SHE'S fat. Or that she's getting fat. Or that she might get fat. Whatever it is, the girl is obsessed about her weight—which, I find out, became a concern after she read up about Seroquel, a medication I prescribed for her agitation, and learned that weight gain is a possible side effect.

The two of us talk in a corner near the nursing station, where she corralled me after her morning group.

"I've also been vomiting my food lately," she says. "I can't help it. I don't want to get fat."

This is an important moment. I don't want to overreact. From a medical standpoint, Linsey appears okay. Her skin turgor is appropriate. She's well hydrated. She doesn't have any hair banding (subtle, alternating, one-inch-long bands from the scalp to the ends of the hair) or other signs of an out-of-control eating disorder. Her vital signs are normal. Her labs are normal. She's been doing well with peers.

"I really want to do what you guys are telling me," she says. "But I'm frightened about my eating. I don't want to take my Seroquel any-more."

"Don't you think it's helping?" I ask.

"Yes, but I'm freaked out it'll make me fat. I've been spitting it out."

Her face is a round pillow of anxiety. I snag Alexi as she walks by and wave the three of us toward the empty examining room. Linsey stares out the window as I bring Alexi up to date on the situation. I don't have to explain my concern. Even with her medical management, Linsey is spitting out her pills and not following directions. This is willful self-sabotage. It's anathema to the process of recovery.

Why? It means her disease is still in charge and dictating her care. It doesn't feel that way to Linsey, of course. She feels scared and in danger. Her brain is telling her to rely on her own devices for survival. *Don't listen. Don't trust anyone, including the doctors, nurses, and counselors.* Why should she trust us when all the important people in her life have violated her trust?

"We're trying to find something to help you with these mood swings and agitation," I say. "I'm going to change your medication from Seroquel to lithium, which shouldn't make you gain any weight."

"But if I do?" she asks.

"We'll try something else."

"What if there's nothing else?" she says in a panicky tone.

"The goal is to get you off everything, and we're almost there," I say, looking intently into her eyes, kicking myself for creating a situation where medication became such a focus for her. "The thing you have to understand is that I'm here for you. Everyone here has your interests in mind. Our job is to support you. But you must trust us and follow our directions. That's it. It's up to you."

"I know, I know," she says.

"Take a breath," I say.

She inhales deeply, and then exhales. Then she does it again.

"I'm a fucking freak," she says. "Oh my God, I can't believe what a frigging mess I am."

Not long after she leaves, Alexi tells me to peek inside the room closest to the nursing station whenever I have time. No hurry. A short time later I look inside the room. Oh my gosh. Our chronic alcoholic, Mitch, is back. He's laying facedown on his bed in a pool of drool. It's disgusting.

"For some reason, I'm more concerned about him this time," says Alexi. "So I put him right next to the nursing station."

"You can see the muscular wasting and the thinning of his skin," I add. "He's too young to look so old and decayed."

"The thing is, he's so smart and funny."

"I know."

Mitch is one of the most frustrating patients I've had. His behavior is the same each time. Once aroused, he slowly pulls himself together, explaining his relapse in a fantastically complicated weaving of bullshit that eventually ends with some sort of excuse about why he relapsed. He blames his father, his boss, his wife. The poor choices he makes never have anything to do with him.

But then the games begin. Although his previous stay was unusually brief, I have a clear recollection of the time before that. After about ten days, I ran into him as he walked to lunch. His hair was well groomed, and he held his broad, chiseled chin up high. His tremor was gone, and his gait was steady. These were all signals that he was through detoxing—which only meant that we were in for his maneuvers.

He started in immediately, telling me that he'd done his second step and his sponsor said he was ready to go.

"Have you arranged a bed in Sober Living?" I asked.

"No, Drew," he said in his usual ingratiating manner. "I don't think I need all that. My dad had to pay for this hospitalization. I'd maxed out my insurance. I'm not about to ask him to pay for Sober Living, too."

"Mitch, how many times are we going to go through this?" I say. "You simply aren't going to get well without adequate treatment.

That's a fact. You've tried it your way how many times? It's time to capitulate and let other people who know what they're doing make some decisions. Right now your diseased brain is calling the shots. You're going to relapse as sure as the two of us are standing here."

Smiling confidently, he put his arm around my shoulder and let me know he had it all figured out. He told me I worried too much, and gave me some mumbo-jumbo about needing faith in the restorative ability of a Higher Power—as called for, he added, in the Big Book. He was referring to the Big Book of AA, which he'd coopted and garbled into something completely inaccurate. Listening to him, I had one thought: *Disaster ahead.* I knew we'd see him again soon.

Alexi reminds me of similar conversations she's had with him in the past. "I don't know how many of these relapses he has in him," she says. "His body is showing the effects."

"It's a progressive disease," I add.

"It's so clear in him," she says. "Each relapse is more intense."

Someone standing on the outside of all this might well ask whether moments like this make me feel I'm not doing my job. Or why anyone should bother with that twelve-step stuff if it doesn't work. Admittedly, sometimes it's so frustrating I can't stand it. I want to strangle someone like Mitch, even though I know better. His game infuriates me. Addiction is the only disease in which people need to be convinced that a) they have a disease and b) they need treatment. With Mitch, I'm at the point where I wonder if we're actually enabling his disease just by letting him use us again and again to piece him back together.

So why bother?

Here's why: Mitch is suffering from a life-threatening disease. So are all the others like him. It's incumbent upon us to find a way to reach these people and offer them the opportunity to get better. No doubt my own codependency keeps me slugging away at cases like Mitch's, perhaps longer than is good for him. But so what? What's the alternative?

And there's another factor at work here, one I find fascinating and poignant: I believe that addiction is a function of evolutionary pressures on populations. And where are the most severe biological burdens of addiction? In populations subjected to repeated genocidal assaults. Addicts tend to be descendants of the people who survive such extreme adversity. They tend to be smarter, more sensitive, and richer human beings. They move the species forward.

But there's a cost, and that's the disease they inherit. If we as a species had never learned how to distill spirits, extract anything narcotic from the poppy, invent benzodiazepines, and so on, these individuals would have a different constitution than the average person—but no disease. The switch in their brains wouldn't get thrown if not for such powerful chemicals. As with any other disease, we have to ask what's causing it and how we treat it.

To me, addiction is the predominant health issue of our time. Abuse, neglect, and abandonment—all are actions that interrupt the healthy development of an individual: These are problems that affect the whole of society. None of us is immune from the resulting problems, which include not only addiction but domestic violence, crime, homelessness, rising health care costs, and above all else individual emptiness.

That's my biggest concern. Our culture has taken its great founding principle, the pursuit of happiness, and twisted it into an obsession with instant gratification, the quick fix, getting what's mine. *Just do it,* indeed: The most successful creative figures in our culture, from the producers of reality TV to the editors of *Maxim* to the directors of music videos, have created an orgiastic mythos of sex, mayhem, and cool clothes. Want to know why spring break kids all act like they're living in one big porn video? Ask the advertisers.

But none of this has anything to do with happiness. In truth, it's just a setup for disappointment, frustration, and failure.

It's why so many people complain about depression, or insist they just don't feel good. Lacking adequate attachments, they feel empty.

They try to feel better by grasping at the solutions the culture offers, only to find that those solutions turn into the problem; then they get caught up in a continued need for arousal, to escape their emptiness.

And even when the evidence of a problem becomes overwhelming, the human capacity for denial can hamper any individual's chances of jumping off the treadmill of addiction. A recovering counselor once told me my favorite story about denial: He came home every night for years completely wasted from drinking, and in the morning his wife complained that he'd been abusive and angry to her. Since he didn't recall a thing, he dismissed this as her problem. Then one morning she placed a tape recorder on the kitchen table and said, "Listen to this." She pushed PLAY and he heard a voice that sounded like him ranting and raving at his wife. Afterward, he was livid. How dare she hire an actor to impersonate him!

Basically, people don't know how they're supposed to feel anymore.

Human beings feel best when they're spending time face to face, particularly in times of adversity or when they're feeling threatened. If nothing else, we learned that from September 11. We define ourselves by the way we relate to other people. We get deep, lasting, and meaningful satisfaction from giving selflessly to, and being present with, others. We develop trust. We feel better about ourselves and our world. This is what we've forgotten: Our decisions should be made on the basis of what's most healthy, not what will satisfy me quickest. *Live with integrity and a clear sense of right and wrong. Consider consequences. Listen to the inner voice of your instinct as carefully as a doctor checks your heartbeat.* This is what I wish we all knew to do.

My patients can't do that. Like so many others, they're struggling with the effects of trauma suffered early in life, when they were still developing the brain mechanisms that allow them to relate to other people and the world in general. Their development was arrested at whatever age the trauma happened. Unable to trust, they grow up without a sense of self. They're overwhelmed by feelings, unable to cope, always out of control.

So where's the doorway out of this hell? Through acceptance of the disease, and through experiencing the pain and the consequences it has caused. The irony is cruel. It's the most vivid part of a patient's reality, and the one they want to most deny. The guilt and shame are profound. Their brains tell them to manage the pain by getting loaded. Then, when they find their way to us, we ask them to go back and *experience* that powerlessness, the very thing that sent them off the rails in the first place.

No wonder they resist.

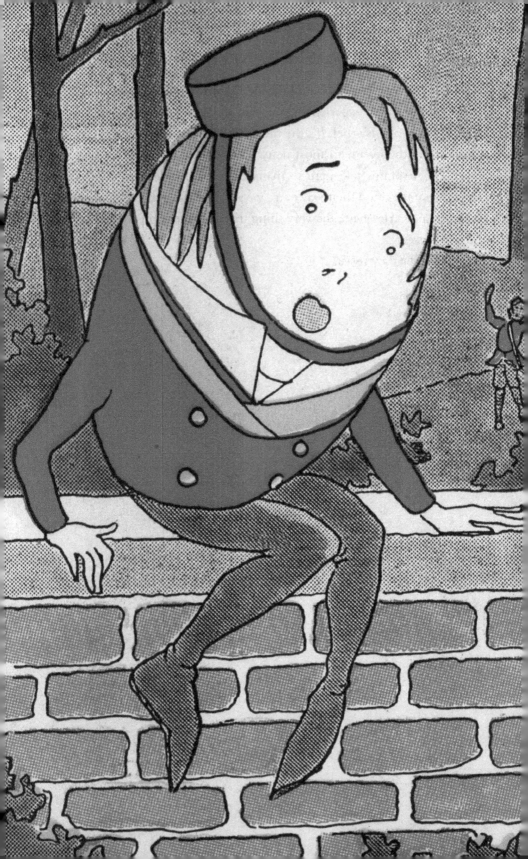

Sixteen

IT'S AFTERNOON. I'M on my way to the treatment team's weekly meeting when I bump into Pat, one of the two counselors, who is also heading toward the conference room. Pat is a talented, compassionate, but imposing recovering heroin addict. Even on hot days he still wears two long-sleeved shirts to cover the tracks and tats that remind him of his disease.

I've just left Amber's room, and as we fall into step together Pat asks, "How's she doing?"

"She's having a tough time coming to terms with her powerlessness," I say.

"She's not the only one, is she?" He gives me a meaningful look. "Aren't you feeling a little frustrated by her yourself?"

"Point taken."

"You've gotta be careful with that one. We have to push her. She can handle it. We have to stop coddling. In fact, as soon as the meeting is done I'm going to review her first step with her to see how it's coming. She's going to keep sliding if we don't stay on top of her."

"I don't know if I agree completely."

"I can see right through her," argues Pat. "I see her working you for meds all the time. She's got so much shit in her. I know what she's about."

I walk into the meeting stunned by his comment. All the principals are already in the room, either seated or standing by the coffeemaker, waiting for a fresh pot. I turn Pat's words over in my mind. He's probably right. Each of us has our own response to patients, after all. I know I'm always taking on everyone else's feelings as if they were my own burden, particularly women's. Amber seems to have found a pathway into that primitive part of my makeup, and that's what Pat has picked up on.

I know this is one of my weaknesses: I can't always catch the complexity of my own reaction to a woman in pain. Of course, that fact itself only makes these meetings more valuable: By sharing our experiences with patients, we sharpen our faculties in debate, catch each other in mistakes, and use our experience in different professional disciplines to make each other better at what we do.

"So where's Matty at?" asks Finley, directing his question to Pat.

"Well, you know, Matty is Matty," he says. "He's self-absorbed, not really interested in sobriety."

"Did he do a first step?"

In our program, the first step, admitting powerlessness, is a requirement; so is getting a sponsor. We'd love to see them get through the second and third steps, too, but that takes weeks, and very few have the resources to cover such a lengthy hospitalization. We give them education and workbooks on the steps.

The goal is to bring about a new awareness of the extent of their disease, its effects on their lives, and the alternatives. Ideally, this leads to opportunities for patients to experience themselves on a new emotional level. If it were all cognitive work, I'd just have to convince them to change their thinking. But the change must be made in the emotional centers of the brain. This is experiential learning, and it takes time—a reality that insurance companies, among others, don't understand.

"Yeah," he nods; Matty took at stab at completing his first step—on the face of it. "But it was just so he could get closer to getting out of here."

"How was it?" asks Finley.

"He was able to identify the consequences, but he still insists that he's not powerless over drugs and alcohol. He kept suggesting he was going to use his will to overcome his drug problem. There was no sense of capitulation to the unmanageability in his life. He remains focused on people, places, and things. He insisted he'd let his boss and his girlfriend get to him—that *that* was why his use had escalated."

"Very superficial," says Finley.

"He doesn't see the biological effects of the drugs," I add.

"He remembers the anxiety and the agitation, but he's got no insight into how manic he was when he came in," says Alexi.

"It's amazing how difficult it is for them to see it," I say.

"Not really," says Pat. "Lest you forget, they're so fucked up they don't know anything."

"Point taken," says Finley.

"He's cooperative," interjects Gail, the other counselor. "I had him earlier today. As a matter of fact, he went ahead and did a second step."

The second step of Alcoholics Anonymous acknowledges belief in a "power greater than ourselves that could restore us to sanity."

"That's ridiculous," says Finley. "We shouldn't have accepted his first step. Don't you think it should've been redone?"

"If you're asking that question, you're going to love this," Gail continues. "He hasn't presented his second step to the group yet, but I went over it with him. He insists his *girlfriend* is his higher power."

The whole room giggles and groans.

"Fantastic," I say. "Get him to redo his first step. Maybe if we can get to some level of honesty, we can deal with his concept of higher power."

Finley leans forward. "Whatever his whim is in the moment—that's his higher power," he says.

For a split second, I imagine what it must be like to be Matty, and I flash on a scene I'd recently witnessed at the airport. A four-year-old boy began crying in the terminal as his mother walked to the ticket counter. He was clearly frightened by the crowd. Immediately, his father, a twenty-three-year-old version of Matty, yanked him close, put his face nose-to-nose against the child's, and in a menacing voice said, "Shut up!"

The little boy cried even harder as his father walked away with him, and I cringed along with him. The boy was crying in the first place because he was feeling anxious and powerless, and instead of getting what he needed from an adult, he got rage, abuse, and separation from his mother—exactly what he feared in the first place.

That's how it happens. Soon there'd be a wall built around his unbearable pain and powerlessness. Soon we'd have another Matty.

Finley picks up another chart, glances at the front page, and shakes his head. "So our friend Mark Mitchell is back," he says. "He'll make us feel better."

Alexi doesn't look up from the papers in front of her. "I'm concerned about him," she says. "He doesn't have many more of these left in him. He's developing muscular wasting. His liver enzymes are way up. He has enlarged red blood cells. His nutrition is horrible. Each time he gets worse. His binges are longer, and his withdrawals are more intense."

"How's he doing now?" asks Finley.

"Finally through withdrawal," she says.

"He was in group this morning," says Debra. "But he was still out of it. He just sat there. Actually, he slept through most of it."

"Enjoy that," cracks Pat. "It won't last. Soon he'll take over."

"It pains me to say it, but I'm not sure this guy's ever going to get better," I say.

"Agreed," continues Pat. "This is his fifth treatment. He never follows through. He always manages to weasel out of our recommendations."

"He went to Sober Living after the last treatment, right?" asks Finley.

"No. Not even close," I answer. "He split when we started pushing him to meet his behavioral goals."

"So unlike him," says Alexi. "That's why I'm worried."

"He went directly to live in the apartment of another patient, a female," I say. "Both of them relapsed."

"He's never capitulated," says Alexi, who turns to the two counselors.

"We need to point out he's never gone beyond the superficial," I say. "He's the kind of guy that, if we could just get him to stay sober long enough to get to a fourth step—"

I notice Finley and Alexi staring at me in disbelief. I stop talking.

"Okay, then," says Finley. "Back to reality."

Sort of. The last point of the meeting is almost beyond belief, too. Linsey has made progress. After hurrying through the details of her medical status—which is stable, including her eating disorder—Pat reports that she did her first step. Since these weekly meetings are my only involvement with a patient's steps, I listen intently for the reaction. Was it honest? Strong? Emotional? Superficial? Complete and accurate? Still romanticizing the life?

My eyes are on Pat, who describes Linsey's delivery as "one of the most powerful steps I've heard in a long time."

"Really," I say. "Good for her. What happened?"

"She sat down with twelve pages on her lap. I thought, oh boy, she's just going to *read* it? We're going to have to push on her to get something out of this. But she sat down and began to read, and poured out so much emotion. She tried to make herself so small in her chair, but she climbed right out of it."

"What were some of the details?" asks Finley.

"She told about going to boarding school at fourteen and discovering pot while hanging out with the kids who did drugs. At a party, she sat next to a guy she thought was cute, a high schooler, and he put his hand up her dress. 'And that was the first time I was raped,' she said. I got a chill."

"And her use escalated after that incident?" I ask.

"Right," says Pat. "God bless her, she didn't leave anything out. Rape. Trading sex for drugs. Abusive relationships with other addicts. Her parents' neglect."

"Beverly Hills is such a nice place to grow up, isn't it?" snickers Alexi.

"You know, before she came here, she was dead," continues Pat. "They revived her at Century City. She discussed her ambivalence at having survived. Now she very much wants to live."

"How'd her peers react?" I ask.

"They gave her terrific feedback."

Good news comes in small increments, but you learn to be grateful for whatever you get. It inspires the whole staff, as well as the patients. It's a phenomenon unique to this sort of medicine. Nowhere else can one patient's successes in recovery have such a profound effect on a group of other patients. They see their disease operating in their peers.

In reality, many patients are so preoccupied by their own shame and suffering that they won't hear a word of a story like Linsey's. But one or two might find themselves so profoundly affected that it helps them find the courage to do their own steps in a genuine and honest manner.

That's how it works. The twelve steps of AA are simply empirical structures that have proved useful for getting addicts to engage slowly in a therapeutic process. Fundamentally, they are a structured journey into a healthy, intimate relationship. There are numerous theories about why addicts are able to connect with one another in this process. Most believe they connect around a common experience of pain and powerlessness without the fear of exploitation. Their pain is so raw and tender that getting them to start the process requires them to be convinced that their pain will be understood. They're all people with extreme trust issues, and the only people they've ever trusted are other addicts. They understand each other. (Interestingly, doctors have discovered that survivors of torture have similar reactions to treatment. They don't open up unless they're around others who've been through similar horrors, as though the pain of being misunderstood would be too great of a risk.)

That's why patients present their steps to their peers. The staff determines whether the step is acceptable, but the real feedback comes from their peers. Sometimes the insights they have are brilliant. They're so attuned to one another's bullshit, they can sniff out a lie before it's halfway uttered. They know when someone's in trouble. They also sense when someone is making progress. Unless you've been through it, you don't know.

Pat reminds me of that point after the meeting. I can't put myself in Amber's shoes and make her do what I want. "It has to come from inside her," says Pat.

"We've had good talks. I thought I sensed her coming around."

"If you ask me, I think you're responding to her pathology. And some very pretty eyes."

"You think I need to pull back?"

"Boundaries, Doctor."

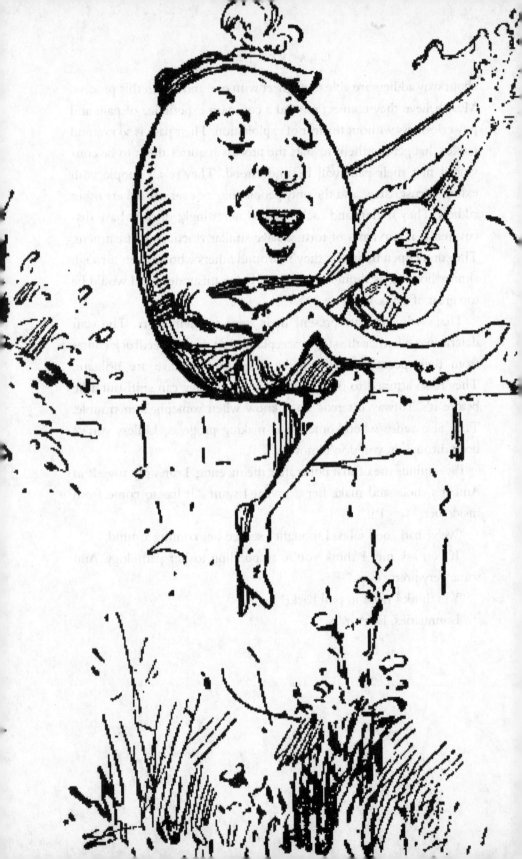

Seventeen

PAT'S COMMENTS MAKE me toss and turn through the night. He's probably right. I'm not perfect. No matter how much I want to care for her, Amber has to navigate the straits and narrows of this disease for herself. She has to summon the strength to pull herself through. Rather than rescue her, which just perpetuates her dependency, my job is to help Amber find a way to manage her feelings and engage in the program.

I stare at the walls all night, hoping to find that clarity within myself. A part like that is easier written than put into practice. At the first sign of daylight, I get out of bed feeling anxious. On my way to work I remind myself to be more vigilant, to pay more attention to my limitations.

I put my hand on the door leading into the unit and take a deep breath. Sometimes I wish I could rearrange my emotions the way I would clothes in my dresser. But I can't. Once inside, everything I vowed to keep in the forefront of my mind blends in with the daily activity; soon I can't even remember a sleepness night, never mind a promise to be more attuned.

"Oh boy, wait till you get a load of this new one," says Alexi, dropping a chart in front of me. "She's wacky."

"I can't wait," I say. "Wacky. Is that a new diagnostic category?"

On the walk to her room, Alexi fills me in about Wendy, a brunette in her mid-twenties. She's a stripper, says Alexi, adding with a wink, "She said she was stripping to make cash so she could go to school."

"Fantastic," I sigh. "Another one with an original plan."

"I wonder if I should start stripping to pay for my daughter's violin lessons?" she says.

Alexi goes on to hint that Wendy's going to be one of those patients whose mere presence will upset the unit's fragile balance of personalities. She's outspoken, given to big gestures and loud outbursts, and sexually provocative, which means that her interaction with male patients will be a problem.

As for her medical problem, Alexi explains, "She's been using Vicodin, taking twenty to thirty pills a day for the last couple months. Prior to that, it was much less. But she's been on it for about a year, ever since a knee injury. There's some question about recent benzos. If so, it was likely an effort to get off the opiates. This all came out when she was caught shoplifting."

"Hmmm," I say, raising my eyebrows.

"I know, it sounds familiar," she says.

"When opiate addicts try to stop, their brains drive them to seek other thrills. Shoplifting is a common manifestation."

"Tell it to the jury," jokes Alexi.

"Pain?" I ask.

"She says it's a ten on the scale. But there's nothing to suggest a source for the pain. She's also complained of hearing loss."

"Interesting," I say. "I saw a report from the Ear Institute that even in normal doses Vicodin can cause hearing loss. Sometimes it's progressive after they stop. So far there's no treatment available for this. Let's watch for that carefully."

Wendy was brought in by a concerned girlfriend after she passed out at a birthday party for the woman's two-year-old daughter. Apparently Wendy had a few drinks—following the shoplifting incident, her drinking probably spiraled out of control—and passed out at the party, hitting her head on the corner of a table. There's a bandage on her forehead; the wound beneath it needed eight stitches. When we enter her room, Wendy is devouring a large bag of M&Ms: she's eating "the greens first," she says, "followed by the blues, and then it doesn't matter."

Her room looks like it's been ravaged by a cyclone. Clothes and belongings are everywhere. On the other hand, she's taken some care to place two personal photographs on her nightstand. One shows her with what I assume is her family, her middle-aged mother and an older brother; the other is of her as a kid at Disneyland. Her idealized self, I imagine.

Wendy no longer resembles that little girl in any significant way. Her tongue is pierced. I notice a couple of tattoos. And fake boobs. She's dressed in a barely-there tank top and low-slung sweat pants that reveal a leopard G-string around her hips. I have a hard time not feeling embarrassed as I look at her. This is how she chooses to relate to others, yet she has no conscious appreciation of how she affects them.

"I know who you are," she says. "Sometimes I listen to you on the radio."

She's already testing the boundaries, trying to manipulate to her advantage. I don't want to give any signals that could be interpreted by her as familiar. I keep Alexi close by while taking a step or two back myself. Suddenly I couldn't be more aware of every thought and action I have. *Be present; don't get sucked in. Just stand there and take down her medical history.*

"When was your last use?" I ask.

"Last night, I think," she says. "Before I passed out."

"Do you remember where you were?"

"At work. I'm a dancer," she says. "My girlfriend was having a birth-day party for her little girl."

"At a club?"

"In the dressing room," she says, and then adds, "I know. It's pretty fucked up for the kid."

To say the least. I glance at Alexi, who makes a note reminding us to investigate a little further, maybe alert Child Services.

"Have you been taking Valium, Xanax, anything like that?"

"I had some Klonopin last week," says Wendy. "And, sure, Xanax whenever it's around."

"How much in the last week?"

"Mostly Klonopin this week," she says. "The blue ones. Maybe six or ten, or, you know, I really can't remember."

When asked about her family's medical history, Wendy paints a loving picture of her mother. Her father, she explains, left when she was nine. There hasn't been much contact since then. He's a druggie, she says, an alcoholic. She also admits that he sexually abused her. She offers some details, but without any trace of emotion. I'm just about able to contain my outrage at the constant outpouring of stories like this; it's all I can do not to lose it front of Wendy, who's only the latest in the long parade of victims who have crossed my path. No doubt her dad was only the first of many perpetrators. In an attempt to regain control and power in her relationship to men, Wendy fetishized her body. The pierced tongue, the fake breasts, the tattoos, the provocative clothes, the job. While she believes she dealt with the abuse long ago, the reality is different: She may not be preoccupied by her memories, but deep-seated feelings about the way she was treated have imprinted themselves on her brain in a way that affects every aspect of how she relates to herself and others.

I ask her to lay down so I can examine her. I also ask Alexi to help—not that I need any, but I have other, obvious reasons.

I work quickly and in silence. It's all about maintaining distance, and yet, as happens with so many female patients, I find myself imagining what kind of horrors were inflicted upon this woman when she was an innocent young girl. Soon I'm agonizing for her. Then Wendy experiences some pain when I press on the lower left quadrant of her abdomen. Upon further questioning, she takes my hand and presses it more firmly into the spot, saying, "Right there."

"Any changes in your period?" I ask.

She shakes her head no. That surprises me. Opiates cause changes in the dopamine levels in the hypothalamus that suppress ovulation.

"Diarrhea? Constipation?"

She shrugs. She must have been somewhat constipated from all the opiates. The diarrhea will hit with the withdrawal.

She's also in pain from withdrawal. She mentions that quite a few times. In general, though, Wendy is in fairly good health. Before leaving her room, I can't resist commenting on her habit of clicking the little barbell in her tongue against her teeth. Since there aren't any rules against it, I can't tell her to stop, but it annoys the hell out of me. "I've seen a ton of chipped teeth from those things," I say.

She shrugs. "I don't get too many complaints from it," she says. "But weren't you going to give me something for the pain?"

I tell Wendy to prepare herself to feel a lot worse before getting better, and not to expect us to be her new drug dealers. She's going to need to start paying attention, and learn to follow the staff's directions. We treat thousands of addicts, I tell her; we know what it takes to get better.

Outside, Alexi rolls her eyes. "Did you see the way she held your hand on her abdomen?" she says. "Oh my God, I thought she was going to pull you right down into bed with her."

"Sorry, I didn't notice," I lie.

"She's a mess," Alexi says. "We've got to get her meds going or she's going to put us through hell."

She does anyway. The rest of the day and on through the next,

Wendy complains in the worst way about excruciating pain in her knee. She calls us every hour till we could set our watch by her. All of a sudden we'll hear her scream, "Holy fucking shit! When are you going to give me something for my goddamn leg?"

Her leg is fine. The opiate withdrawal is her problem. Despite the medication we're giving her, she's still in terrible pain. Everyone knows it, too. They can't help but know it. Wendy makes sure everyone knows she's miserable. Some patients burrow into an invisible hole as they go through withdrawal, hiding under the covers in their beds, their drapes pulled down and the lights off. They want to be left alone.

Not Wendy, who is dramatic, expansive, and intrusive.

On her third day in the unit, she has managed to burn out Alexi. "I've had enough," she says upon seeing me that day.

"What do you mean?"

"Follow me," she says. "Let's go."

She takes me to Wendy's room and we walk in. Wendy is on her bed, holding onto the headboard while raising her torso and legs straight into the air. Total exhibitionism, total ridiculousness. Groaning, she says, "This is the only way I can be comfortable." I look at Alexi and the two of us crack up. Neither of us comments, though. "Come on, Wendy, let's go to group," I say. "Get your mind off the pain."

Amber is affected by Wendy's behavior. As I am about to leave, she asks if she can speak to me for a moment. At first, she asks how Wendy is doing. A patient as brittle as Amber would much rather focus on someone else's pain. But it's hard. With her empty emotional landscape, she's easily invaded by other people's intense feelings. Still, I encourage her to focus on her own treatment.

"But did you notice that girl's eyes?" she asks.

Yes, I have. "What about them?" I ask.

"They're wild and crazy," she says.

"Kaleidoscopic is the word that occurs to me," I say.

"Am I as fucked up as she is?" she asks.

I nod and raise my shoulders, metabolizing that reality for her and reflecting it back in a way she can tolerate. If she could read my eyes, they'd say, "This is a bad disease you have." She takes something from me that allows her to continue reflecting on Wendy.

"I don't even remember coming here," she says. "Isn't that freakish?"

"Not really," I say. "Most patients go through such intense withdrawal that they don't remember their first few days or even the whole first week."

"I remember feeling like shit," she says. "I still feel like shit. But I remember being hit by wave after wave of pain." Amber looks up at me with big eyes awash in tears. Given her typical disconnect and periodic dissociative flashbacks, it's a rare moment of real connection for her. My instinct is to hug her, the way it would be for any caring person, but that would cross the very boundaries I'm trying to define with Amber. Instead I compliment her on getting through the worst of her withdrawal, and on embracing her feelings. I tell her I'm proud of her strength, and I urge her to share that story in her next group.

Later, I find I'm still thinking about that encounter. You never know for sure, but I believe Amber and I had one of those significant moments when a patient takes a completely honest look at their past, present, and future, and decides—maybe without knowing or articulating it—to reconnect with humanity after years of being cut off. If her recovery happens, she'll need years to get entrenched and feel the full effect. It was one brief moment in which she allowed herself to accept connectedness and experience herself as reflected by another person. She will need thousands more such moments, and with luck they'll happen between her and her sponsor, and with her peers.

I won't be a part of that process. But I love being present for the moment it all turns around.

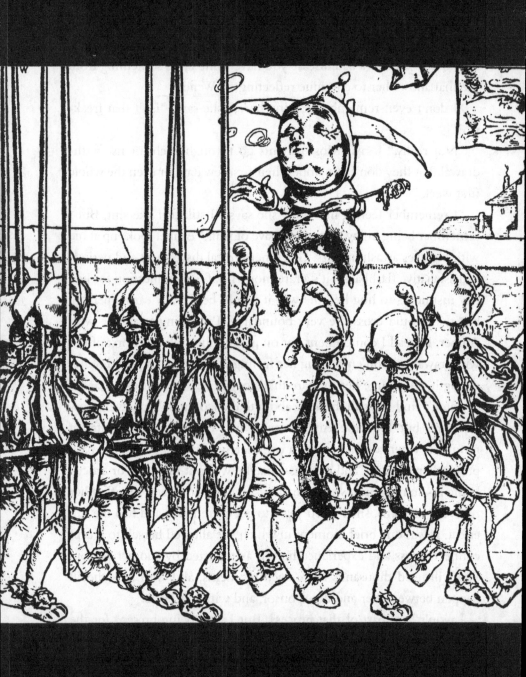

Eighteen

"HOW'D IT HAPPEN?" I ask. "One minute two patients are here, and the next they're gone. Who was doing the accounting? Who saw them last?"

It's the next day, and Wendy and Matty have disappeared from the unit. I gather the staff, and they know I'm upset. According to everyone's recollection, Wendy and Matty were at breakfast and attended morning group. They also ate lunch and had a smoke on the patio, where apparently they spoke to each other one-on-one for the first time.

Though Wendy hasn't caused any problems for us since being admitted roughly four days earlier, we take her disappearance as a serious health risk. Even at her best she's unable to control her impulses, and she's hardly at her best. In the throes of withdrawal, she's in danger of hurting herself. Of course she's not legally bound to stay at the hospital, but if she's here we're obligated to make an effort to find her and keep her safe.

I double-check Wendy's room. It's empty. I glance around quickly. The room is as messy as it was when I was in there the day before. I open the closet, in case she's hung herself and nobody's thought to look. I'm not being morbid. Since most patients suffer severe depression during withdrawal, all have to be considered suicide risks. It wouldn't be out of the question for someone with Wendy's issues. Fortunately her closet is empty, except for a pair of men's flip-flops that must've belonged to a previous patient.

Before I close the door again, though, I notice a window in the back of the closet. I guess it's left over from the last remodel. The view is of the back ninety, our nickname for the large stretch of undeveloped chaparral behind the hospital. A hazard of dirt, brush, and trees, it's our danger zone. We regularly catch patients out there either using or scoring drugs. Now, with the sun starting its descent in the west, it's a field of light and shadows. I scour the scene intently, and after a few minutes I see something move. Maybe not. I try to focus on the spot, but I can't tell for sure. *Shit.*

Darting out the door in the adjacent room, I scramble across the dirt. About twenty-five yards out, I hear the sound of a man's voice. A second later, a woman's gentle laugh helps me narrow my search. I wonder if they're smoking grass or trading hits off a crack pipe. Then I see Wendy and Matty. He's naked. She's still wearing her tank top. They're having sex.

What happened to Wendy's knee pain? Did it suddenly clear up?

No, she merely discovered that sexual arousal gratifies her addictive biology the same way drugs do. She wasn't able to stop herself, wasn't able to manage her feelings. Her addict brain had taken over. The temporary relief it provides is enough to get her through the moment. The act is also something she has relied on for validation her whole adult life. Losing herself with someone she perceives as a powerful male makes her feel safe, though ultimately she chooses men who reenact traumatizations and reinforce her shame, guilt, and her sense of herself as a victim.

I shout at Wendy and Matty, telling them to get dressed and meet me in their rooms. Then I return to the unit and let everyone know I found them.

Everyone knows Matty and Wendy fucked up. The two of them also know they violated their treatment contracts. We don't try to keep the incident quiet. The gossip grapevine among patients in a chemical dependency unit is spectacularly lively. Within minutes, all the patients knew what had happened.

The counselors deflect the buzz by reminding patients of the behavioral contracts they all signed. They drive home the point by reviewing them again.

Alexi can't contain her amusement. "These people are too much," she says.

"So smart, yet so dumb," I say. "Just proves how much they're in the grip of this thing."

They may be powerless, but we aren't. Both Wendy and Matty have to be dealt with—separately, of course. First, though, I want to prescribe some postcoital contraception for Wendy.

"To my knowledge, she's not on birth control," says Alexi.

"If the pharmacy has it, I'd prefer the levonorgestrel-ethinyl estradiol combination," I say. "Two pills now. Repeat them in twelve hours."

"Okay."

"Also, please debrief Wendy and see if she feels in any way that she was coerced into this encounter. If so, we'll have to send her to the ER for a forensic exam. You should also explain to her that postcoital contraception prevents her from ovulating. It's not an abortion. If she's ovulated within the last twenty-four hours, in all probability this won't work and she'll still get pregnant."

"What about Brad Pitt?"

"I'll take care of Matty," I say.

Having followed instructions, he is waiting for me in his room. His roommate, an alcoholic in his fifties nearing the end of his stay, is out. Matty is a big, competitive guy. In such situations, it's usually prudent to bring a nurse into the room, too. I didn't. I don't know Matty well enough to anticipate his reaction. I don't like such confrontations, so I keep my talk short and to the point.

"We try to be a supportive program," I say. "I'd like to give you a chance to come clean with us."

"What?"

"Have you been doing any drugs this morning?"

"No," he says.

"What's your sober date?"

"Eight days," he says.

"Nothing since then?"

"No."

Matty tosses a little piece of paper he's been playing with into the trash can, and gestures like an NBA player when it goes in.

"What's the big deal?" he says.

Irritated, I open his chart and take out his treatment contract. I make sure he sees his signature, and then I point to a paragraph midway down the page. It's the paragraph that explains that sexual contact between patients is not permitted, and furthermore is grounds for discharge.

"Do you recall that?" I ask.

"I thought that meant, like, *rape*," he says. "That chick was really into it."

Matty has to go. If I had any doubt, his last comment erases it. He hasn't gone to groups regularly, another violation of his contract. His constant flirtations with women on the patio have stirred up the other patients. Now this incident. He's toxic, a danger to other patients. We don't have enough structure to contain him.

I tell him that it's not working out. "Let us help you transfer to a more structured unit," I say.

After hearing that, Matty finally gets what's happening, and he reacts in the way I feared. I can see him literally wrestling with a buildup of stress. He starts to argue, listing the ways the program is helping him. Matty's not the kind of guy who wants to be told anything. It triggers his feelings of helplessness, and makes him feel out of control. He can't handle that. It triggers aggressive feelings that guys like Matty can't regulate. I know what's coming.

"Matty, you've got to call your girlfriend or your mother and have one of them pick you up," I say. "We'll give you referrals to Cry Help, Impact House, or another excellent facility."

He slams his fist into a pillow. "I'm paying cash for this program," he says. "I put down five thousand dollars, and I've gotten lousy care. You guys haven't done shit for me. I haven't seen a doctor. You don't give me enough medication. I keep telling you I need more. This morning Alexi wouldn't listen when I told her about my back pain. This is some kind of a ripoff. How much of that money I'm paying goes to you?"

After that outburst, I tell him to make his phone call and then I leave. As I leave I hear him throw something, probably a book, against the wall and scream, "This is *bullshit!* You can't discharge me. I haven't done anything. I'm calling Patient's Rights."

Perfect.

I'm for watchdog organizations like Patient's Rights, but in practice they can end up empowering the most manipulative and disruptive patients. Generally, Patient's Rights assumes a patient is right and the caretaker is wrong. Our only defense is impeccable documentation. It seems we're always filling out forms. Since there's never enough time to complete all the paperwork, patients like Matty may get their way, to their own detriment.

In progressive states like California, patients aren't obliged to follow their doctors' instructions, the rationale being that to force them to do so would infringe on their rights. It's against the law for me even to suggest that we might stop him from calling Patient's Rights. It's like a criminal suspect asking for a lawyer. In fact, if he wants to, I have to *offer* him the opportunity to call. Matty's behavior has been so outrageous that I want to believe even Patient's Rights would see through him. But if he wants to pick up the phone, hey, I can't stop him.

I end up triggering a silent code, an alarm that gathers staff from throughout the hospital to provide a show of force to a patient who is or might become violent. This is as opposed to a more urgent Code White, which is an emergency call for help issued over the entire hospital through the P.A. system, a call for help with a patient who is an imminent danger and must be immediately restrained.

Within seconds of my silent alarm, staff convenes by the nursing station. I'm especially grateful to see the half-dozen large males who show up. The group, about fifteen strong, follows me into Matty's room. Bewildered by the show of overwhelming force, he asks if this is an intervention. In a way it is, I tell him, except the upshot is that he must leave the premises.

"Give him referrals to Cry Help and Impact House," I tell Alexi. "Let him use the phone in the consultation office. If he doesn't want to set up a bed at one of those facilities, have security escort him off the grounds. He needs something more structured. And long-term. Six to twelve months minimum."

About two hours later I pass him in the hall, tell him he has what it takes to get better if that's what he wants. He mutters something about being a New Yorker and being misunderstood. Of course, it's all out there, nothing that he is responsible for. "I don't need any of the bull-shit anyway," he says. And that's the last I see of him.

Meanwhile, Wendy is in her room and falling apart. Alexi has already spoken to her and reported back to me. She had a nurse help Wendy clean herself up after her romp in the dirt. She doesn't know how much of Wendy's response is dramatic effect and how much is real.

"We're just four days into it with her," says Alexi. "This girl is like dead rats in the window."

"What?"

"It's Slav." She laughs. "No matter how nice the merchandise in the store, if you see dead rats in the window it tells you what's really going on."

I take a deep breath before going into Wendy's room. Laying on the bed, her face buried in her pillow, she's still sobbing hard. I notice she's turned down the photos on her nightstand. After talking a bit, she sits up and apologizes. She couldn't control herself, she says, and I know that part is true. Unlike Matty, she seems to be taking some responsibility. Then again, she could also be playing me. I don't know.

"I want to get better," she says. "I don't like living like this. I don't want to go on spending every minute thinking about where and how I'm going to score my drugs. I fucked up. I don't know why I do these things. I know they aren't right. I need help. Please let me stay."

"How many second chances have you asked for?"

"I don't know," she cries. "Too many."

"In order for me to let you stay here, you have to be willing to follow all the rules to the letter," I say.

"I will. I swear."

I hand her a brand-new treatment contract, containing additional and more rigid restrictions, and tell her to read it carefully.

"All the rules are right there in black and white," I say. "We'll be holding you accountable for everything. If you have questions you should ask them now, because telling me later on that you didn't understand won't work."

Wendy nods. Still, no matter what I tell her, I suspect we're going to have more problems ahead. If she's going to have a chance, she needs help dealing with her impulses. I restrict her to the unit. She appears to accept the news well. She doesn't argue. Nor does she balk when I tell her that she can't abuse the staff, have any inappropriate contact with her peers, or miss any groups.

"I also expect you to *participate* in group," I say. Group, I explain, might allow her access to the emotional material that's driving her need to escape. "No more bullshit. Be on time to all groups—no exceptions."

I sound like a teenager's parent. Of course, she's acting like a teenager. This is a lot of information for her to absorb. I know three-quarters of it passes right through her, untouched and undigested. But part of my job is to repeat it over and over again until something does stick.

A little later I get concerned and check on her. Call it a bad premonition. Luckily, it's nothing. Though still in her room, Wendy is calmer. I don't know what kind of issues she might have regarding family or insurance, but I sense that she's scared. Part of her doesn't want to blow it, and part of her simply doesn't know how to be anything but out of control, and yet inside she's a cauldron of roiling emotions. "I know you feel shame," I say.

She's silent; she looks right at me, but I notice a cold emptiness to her eyes. She is struggling with the powerlessness over her disease and the shame this creates. And she's dealing with it in the only way she has ever known—by dissociating from her feelings. This is her escape when there is no escape.

Dissociation is the activation of a primitive region of the brain that we share with lower life forms. It's basically the remnant of the mechanism that's responsible for an animal's feigning death when threatened. In this state, Wendy is reliant on behaviors like sex or drug use for relief from her feelings. The look in her eyes sets off a cold chill in my spine. I feel a need to reach her.

"The shame sets off a domino effect inside you that ends in catastrophe," I continue. "Trust me, feeling your feelings won't destroy you. You might feel helpless right now, but you aren't helpless. If you were helpless, you wouldn't be at this facility. We're all here to help you. We know what works, and your job is to follow directions. It's time to listen."

"I have too much in my head to listen," she says. "You talk about feelings, but I don't know what I'm feeling."

"You're feeling intense anxiety," I say. "Fear. You don't want to use, and yet your brain is saying you won't be able to manage if you don't use."

She grits her teeth and growls. It's the sound of frustration. "What's going on?" she sobs.

I turn over the two photographs Wendy had placed facedown. Once again the little girl in the two pictures is smiling into the room. Wendy steals a glance and then lays down on the bed, pulling a cover over her and shutting her eyes. I know she's probably lied to me, but when she wakes up she'll see that the person she's hurting most is the one looking back at her, and maybe then she'll start getting the message.

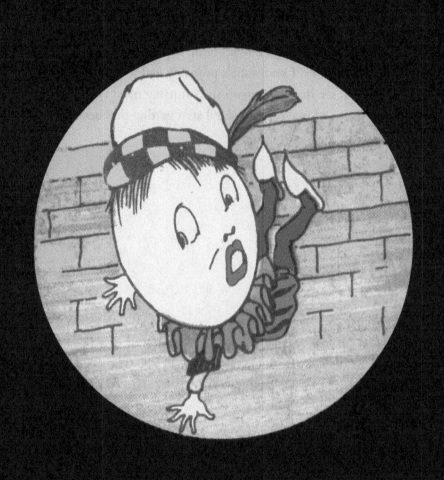

Nineteen

NOT EVERYONE GETS a break.

I'm examining Amber. She should be feeling stronger than she seems to be, and so I'm looking for clues.

"Breathe in," I say. "Deep."

That sounds clear. I move the stethoscope slightly across Amber's back.

"Now breathe normally."

Believe it or not, performing this basic procedure on a survivor of sexual abuse makes me feel awkward. I'm extremely conscious of my movements. Amber is oblivious. She has no idea of my concerns. Still, the slightest misattunement on my part can activate the rage of victimization. Sometimes I behave much more cautiously than required, because I'm especially sympathetic to her pain.

The exam starts out as routinely as the others I've given her over the past three weeks. Nothing out of the ordinary. Then, however, I hear a sound between S1 and S2. It's a faint *whoosh,* the sound of a mid-systolic heart murmur. Hmmm. I ask her to take a few more breaths while I double- and triple-check myself. The sound is unmistakable.

After telling Amber to pull the back of her shirt down, I step around so I'm facing her. She has yet to come out of her shell, but there's something about her now, something I can sense, that lets me know life is returning to her. It is in her eyes. Dante wrote about this, the phenomenon of seeing God reflected in the eyes of Beatrice. To me it's a matter of light and dark, life and death.

Does that sound corny? So what? What's supposed to nourish my soul and sense of purpose more than reaching across the divide and connecting with another human being who hasn't been able to do it alone? What's more satisfying than this flash, this vision, this warm glimpse at the unknowable?

I stare at Amber. For all I saw and felt in that fiery moment, I'm no better than I was before. Neither is she. In fact Amber might be in more precarious territory.

"Has anyone ever said anything to you about a heart murmur?" I ask.

"What?" she asks.

"A heart murmur. Has anyone ever mentioned that? Or mitral valve prolapse?"

"No." She shakes her head slowly.

I see the concern in her face. That's a problem. She's unable to deal with such anxiety. Her brain is sending messages that overwhelm her. Even though she's shrinking right before my eyes, I have to keep going. My job is to steady and stabilize her, as I continue to ask unsettling questions.

"Well, I do get these things in my chest," she adds.

My first thought is, *No, that's not what I mean.* I'm talking about a sound that I hear. But then I remind myself that she's a cocaine addict. She's done a lot of coke. It wouldn't be the first time I've seen a young person with heart damage from cocaine. Coke restricts the blood supply to the heart, dissolving the cordlike fibers that tack down the valves. If the cords break, the valves flap.

"Have you ever had chest pain?" I ask.

"Sometimes. When I'd do a lot of coke, sometimes I would feel like my heart was going to explode inside my chest."

Every addict who's done stimulants has felt that at one time or another. That isn't helping me.

"I'm hearing a turbulent blood flow in your heart," I say. "It doesn't necessarily mean anything. You were a little anemic when you came here. Sometimes anemia can cause a murmur. Many other common conditions can cause murmurs. I don't want you to worry. But I want to look into it further."

She seems to accept this. I order an electrocardiogram for Amber, and I also want to get an echocardiogram. One of these tests looks at how the heart muscle conducts electricity; the other uses sound waves to take an actual picture of the heart. Together they should answer my questions.

I have still another one, though. I don't like the look in Amber's eyes—the glaze, the lifelessness, the cold, opaque appearance that's the opposite of the sparkle of connection. I try making a little light conversation as a way of gently taking her emotional temperature, and this seems slowly to draw her out. Finally she admits, "I keep having these damn panic attacks. Everyone keeps telling me that I'm doing good, but it's too hard. I feel like shit. Nothing's working."

"You need to stay open to the staff and your peers," I say. "That's the only way you'll be able to start managing your feelings."

I leave Alexi in Amber's room to watch for any signs of a postexam panic attack. There's no telling how much more anxious Amber might become once she's left alone. I'm worried, too, and I want those tests scheduled as soon as possible. I ask Julie, the utilization and review nurse in charge of negotiating coverage with insurance companies, to get approval for Amber's electro- and echocardiograms. Already over-burdened, Julie rolls her eyes as if to say, "Sure, I'll get right on it—as soon as I take care of the other ten million problems on my desk."

A few hours later, I find Julie in hell. Actually, she's in her office, but she's got two phone lines going and she's writing furiously on a legal pad. Seeing me in the doorway, she shakes her head no. The poor woman. She has a frustrating, thankless, and absolutely vital job dealing with insurance companies, unraveling red tape, and persuading nurses and clerks two thousand miles away that patients are really sick and need more treatment. It happens with nearly every patient.

She looks relieved when I ask her about Amber. The brightness in her eyes tell me she has an answer, and I'm right. But it's not good news.

"They're going to cover her, but only for two more days," she says.

From her look, I know I'm supposed to infer that she fought for the best coverage she could, and that this is their final response. I find that infuriating. Julie apologizes. It's not her fault, I know. She's as fiercely committed to the patients as anyone. She gets to know all of them and feels terrible when she can't get the responses I want. But she doesn't make the decisions. Nor do I. What we think the patients need has little to do with the reality of what the patients can get.

That falls to the system.

The reviewers she speaks to are generally hostile, hurried, and unsympathetic to the human side of medicine. They want patients in and out as inexpensively as possible.

I know how the conversation went between Julie and the carrier.

Is she eating?

Yes.

Is she walking?

Yes.

Blood pressure okay?

Normal.

What medication is she on? Does she have a place to go? Fine, she's got two more days.

They ignore the fact that she's fragmented, suffering flashbacks and panic attacks, so fragile she knows she'll never make it after she returns to her abusive husband.

But the doctor wants to keep her, argues Julie.

Well, he'll have to talk about that with our doctor.

Nine times out of ten, the results are unchanged. Their decisions are couched in jargon and euphemisms: "Unless you can provide us with more information to substantiate continued inpatient hospitalization," we hear time and again, "we'll be unable to certify any further inpatient days based on our clinical criteria for continued inpatient treatment."

Most insurance policies allow for thirty days of inpatient coverage for chemical dependency, but customers don't know that their carriers sell the policies to review agencies, businesses that make their money by limiting access to coverage. In other words, the less money spent on treating a patient, the more money made by the review agency. What's the motivation for giving someone the best care? Or the care they need? Not as much as one would like to believe.

One day I got a call from a carrier telling me to get rid of a patient who'd been in the unit just three days. A tall, nice-looking black man, he was a severe cocaine addict. After years of addiction, he'd finally checked himself into rehab. It was the first time he'd sought help. Though his withdrawal was very difficult and he was overwhelmed by anxiety and cravings, he really wanted to be there. He'd lost his home, his wife, his job—everything but the thirty days of coverage he had left on his plan.

Then he lost that, too. According to his carrier, there was nothing wrong with him. It didn't matter how vehemently Julie argued.

Having already declared him medically stable, they'd made a decision. They wanted him moved to a residential facility they had on a list. They went so far as to arrange the transfer for the next morning.

That pushed me over the edge. It was the equivalent of me calling another hospital and changing the treatment for a surgical patient without speaking to the surgeon. They also missed another, more subtle issue. This patient was emotionally fragile, with no support system outside the hospital to turn to. He'd made a connection with us. Dismissal at that point would be just another abandonment for him. He might start using again as a result. Or he might decide that no one was worth trusting, which would make it that much more difficult to enroll him in treatment.

It was the most unethical behavior I had witnessed. I called the California State Insurance Commissioner, intending to launch a complaint. Instead I was literally overwhelmed by all the different ways they had for customers to lodge complaints against their HMOs, doctors, nurses, hospitals, and so on. In the process, though, I discovered that they had no protocol for a practitioner who wanted to file a complaint against an insurance company. After hours on the phone, a sympathetic clerk suggested I call my congressman.

In the end, I wrangled another day out of the carrier, a miracle that allowed me to prepare the patient for his transfer, but I never heard from him again.

Unless Julie is able to do something, I fear the same will happen with Amber. She is likely to start using again soon after discharge. I ask Julie to go back and request additional tests, the echo especially. I need that test. Maybe a psychiatric consultation, too. See if they'll agree to that, and prolonged care. I have to keep Amber from leaving.

Julie lets me go through all my explanations without saying a word. She gets it. I know. She does this all day long.

"I'll try," she says. "But don't get your hopes up."

"Please."

"You don't have to beg me. I'm not the problem."

A while later Julie stands before me, perfectly still, with defeat etched across her face. The tests aren't going to happen. Neither is the consult.

I kick my toe into the floor out of frustration. "This woman needs those tests as soon as possible," I say.

"I talked to the reviewer, and they want her out," she says. "According to them, her detox is completed. Her vitals are stable. She needs to step down to outpatient, and then she can see her primary care provider. He can order the echo and the electrocardiogram."

"Listen, she's a cocaine addict," I say. "She's got a new murmur. And I have a funny feeling about it."

Julie shakes her head and says, "You're going to have to give me more than a funny feeling before I can call them back."

It's maddening. Here I know exactly what to do as a doctor, and yet I'm being told I can't do it. I'm left fluttering in the wind, feeling as out of control and powerless as my patients. But as much I'm disturbed, I handle it. That's the difference. I stay focused on work and devote time to my family. In fact, on days like this, it's a relief to drive away and coach my sons' sports teams.

I need that replenishment. Oddly, I don't share much about work with my wife. I'm able to compartmentalize the different parts of my day. I also know that Susan's response to the tales of frustration I'd bring to the dinner table nightly would be to ask, "Why do you care so much? Does anyone else put themselves out that way?"

I can't help but care. I wouldn't know how to hold myself back. My patients are struggling for their very survival, confronting core issues like abuse, neglect, pain, self-esteem, and the absence of love. If I can be their bridge over all that, I'm doing my job. Even if I fail, at least I'm trying. This is why I get so crazed when insurance companies make decisions based on actuarial tables rather than sound, practical medicine.

Early the next day I ask Julie to arrange a doctor-to-doctor review, which is a call between the carrier's physician and me. By their nature, such conversations are rarely pleasant. Nor are they often fruitful. Usually they mean speaking to a doctor in an office in Connecticut for whom revising a decision would mean taking heat from the insurance company, who employs him to get patients out while minimizing any exposure to liability. Translation: They want the patient out ASAP, without making them look bad if something should go wrong.

We never tell a patient their insurance company wants them out. If the carrier heard a hint of that, they'd refer their business elsewhere. We end up using the same stupid euphemisms as the carrier: "Your resources have been exhausted, and we have to find another way to optimize those resources your insurance company has available."

It's a tricky dance that almost always makes me uncomfortable. The few times awful things have happened as a result, I have had insurance companies defend their decisions by saying, "Well, Doctor, it's your signature on the chart discharging the patient. We don't practice medicine."

I don't want to go through that with Amber.

While worrying about her, I'm confronted by someone who doesn't appear to have any worries: Mitch, the alcoholic. He is back. Not only has he risen from the dead, he's taken over the groups, dominating them with his self-absorbed commentary and savvy about the program from having been through rehab enough times.

"He holds court like some sort of senior statesman," says Alexi.

"It's all a defense to deflect anyone from focusing on his issues," I say.

"You should've heard this last meeting," she says. "This young woman, Zona—she's in the outpatient program and still in Sober Living—"

"Yeah, I remember her. Married to a cop. Sexual abuse in her background."

"Right. In group, she was complaining that her husband had

become abusive on the phone. He complained about the stress of managing their house and two children without her."

"Obviously he senses that she's growing away from him as she grows in the program, and he was lashing out," I interject.

"Mitch immediately stood up and launched into a diatribe about the importance of making sobriety a priority in one's life. He told her, 'Your husband needs to support your sobriety. That's *it* right now.' And then he said, 'All of us love you. The Big Book says the codependent is sicker than us. My girlfriend tried to get me to change my sponsor because she didn't like him.' And he just went on and on. It was *always* about him, full of all those twisted references to the Big Book. He sounds like one of those wild TV evangelists."

At that point, Julie bolts into the nursing station and interrupts our conversation. She has the doctor from Amber's insurance company on the phone. She rolls her eyes. That tells me two things: The doctor isn't pleasant, so don't count on anything, and also don't keep him waiting. I don't waste a second.

"This is Dr. Green," he says.

We exchange a couple quick pleasantries, and then I get into the case.

"This is a poly-drug–addicted female in her late twenties with a new cardiac murmur," I say. "She was anemic on admitting labs, but I don't think that explains what I'm hearing. The quality of the murmur suggests to me the possibility of a blown mitral leaflet."

"We're not the medical carrier," he interrupts. "If this is a medical problem, it will have to be referred to her primary care provider."

"I understand," I say. "But this woman needs further inpatient treatment for her chemical dependency. She's extremely labile. She's having intense cravings. She's suffering flashbacks. She's a trauma survivor with profound PTSD. She needs a very high degree of structure, supervision, and support. At this moment, her relapse potential has to approach one hundred percent. In spite of the severity of her condition, she's shown remarkable progress in treatment. I'm convinced that sending her to a medical facility at this point in her treatment would be destabilizing."

He asks for more facts. I describe her vitals, and list the medication we've given her. After a brief silence, he says she sounds stable, and asks me for the basis of continued inpatient treatment. Hasn't he heard what I've said? It doesn't sound like he has. It's very discouraging. Actually, it's worse.

"Dr. Pinsky, we base the need for continued inpatient hospitalization on the published guidelines of the American Society of Addiction Medicine. Your patient does not meet any of our criteria for continued inpatient treatment."

Great. I'm talking about a living, breathing, suffering, pain-riddled human being down the hall who wants to get better but needs help, and he's looking at published guidelines that are open to interpretation. A body versus a black-and-white chart: Where would you go looking for the truth? I remember the first conversation I ever had with such a reviewer. He was a physician for a new local managed care company. He called after one of his "lives," as he referred to her, had checked into our program for the third time in two months. He wanted her out in three days. When I argued that the patient would relapse and lose her job, he said that was precisely his point. She'd lose her job—and her insurance. Then she was no longer their concern.

The rest of our conversation was chilling.

"She might also lose her life," I said.

"I'm an insurance administrator, not a social agency," he replied. "I can't tell you whether that's good or bad."

Now, with Dr. Green, I'm getting the same feeling again. My expertise means nothing. Forget about proper medicine. What about simply helping a human being?

"I'm sorry, Doctor," he says with a tone of condescension. "If you could provide more information, it might be different. But based on what you've told me so far, I can't certify any more inpatient days. She'll need to step down to intensive outpatient."

"Does she have coverage for Sober Living?" I ask.

"I can't tell you that," he says. "I don't have any information about her insurance policy. We're just the review agency."

That's it. After hanging up, I take a walk outside to cool off. When I return to the unit, I still need to vent. I find Alexi, who's discussing something with Finley. Both shake their heads as I recount the conversation. All three of us know a bad decision's been made, and yet we can't do a thing about it. Such is reality. Life is often a series of problems. You get bad news, and then you deal with it.

"She's going to be gone in a day and a half," I say finally. "I'd love to see what's going on before she leaves. Can we at least call Medical Services and see if they can get in touch with her PCP and get approval for the echo and the EKG?"

"They did the EKG about forty-five minutes ago," says Alexi.

"Who ordered it?" I ask.

"I don't know," she says with a wink.

A moment later, I get the results from her chart. They indicate a fast pulse, a slight widening of the QRS complex, and some very wide premature beats that still look atrial, nonspecific changes of the ST/T segments that could represent a restriction of blood to the heart muscle, but don't necessarily. Nothing that specifically suggests trouble. So what about the damn murmur?

I start to second-guess myself. Did I really hear that *whoosh?*

Wait a minute. I look at the EKG results again, and notice something else: Her QT interval might be a little prolonged. It's subtle. Although the computer readout says it corrects to normal, it definitely appears longish. I won't rule out anything. Having recently read a report that raised questions about a possible relationship between the new antipsychotics like Seroquel and QT prolongation with sudden cardiac death, this could be an issue.

I close the folder and turn to Alexi. Her eyes ask, "Well?"

"I don't know," I say. "All this does is continue to worry me."

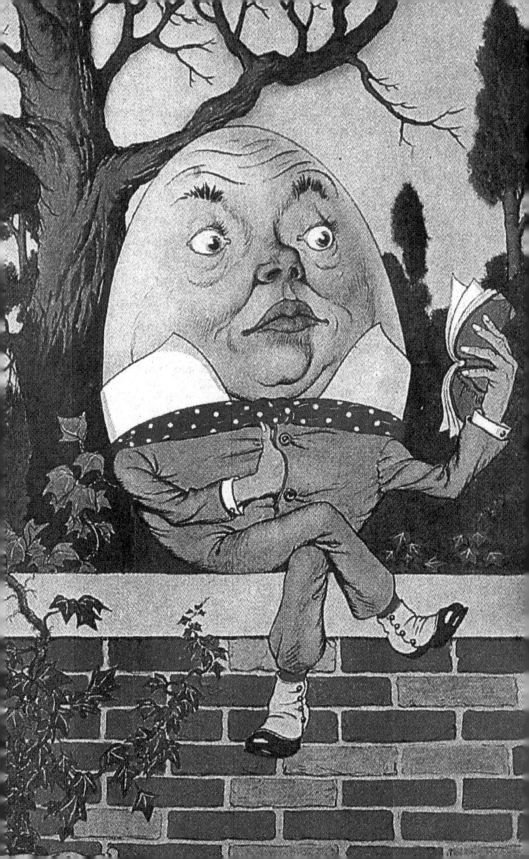

Twenty

UNFORTUNATELY, AFTER ALL my attention to Amber, I'm in New York when she is finally discharged two days later. The timing was beyond my control. I had taken one day off to watch my daughter in an ice skating competition and help coach my boys on the ball field. Then I flew back east for a commitment on *Good Morning America*. While there I opened an e-mail from Alexi updating me on the day's activity in the unit, and saw that Amber had left.

I e-mailed her back, asking for more information. Her response contained some unsettling details: Amber had been picked up by her husband, who said he was taking her to Sober Living, but she hadn't checked in when Alexi called a few hours later. Neither was she there when Alexi called later that night.

Ugh. Reading this stirs all sorts of feelings in me, none of them good. Why couldn't I have done more?

All of a sudden it seems as if I'll be swallowed up by my hotel room walls if I don't leave the building immediately. I need air and space. I end up taking a long walk. There's no better place to lose yourself than the streets of New York City. By the afternoon I'm downtown, in roughly the same place I was about two weeks after the September 11 attacks against the World Trade Center and the Pentagon.

I remember that night. It was a Sunday, and I was walking around Greenwich Village. I was relieved to see the cafés full of people. I'd watched the attacks from three thousand miles away, but as soon as I'd arrived in the city I was on the streets, drawn by a need to participate in the healing process. I began in midtown and went to Ground Zero. I walked for hours, eager just to be around New Yorkers, who managed the trauma by talking and connecting with each other.

I wish I had that same feeling now, as I walk around thinking about Amber. I'm hard on myself at the best of times, and this might be one of the worst. One of the tenets of AA's twelve steps is a spiritual awakening, a belief in a higher power, a general faith that life will work out the way it's supposed to. When I run outdoors in the canyons near my home, I can sometimes connect with something greater than myself and give myself over to it. That's my sense of spirituality.

But I struggle with the concept of faith. How can I have faith when every day I'm confronted by people in pain? How can I have faith when the system can be so coldhearted to someone as clearly in need as Amber? How can I have faith when I failed to help her improve? And if I struggle like this, it's that much harder for my patients. They have a right to ask where God was when such horrible things happened to them. Why should they have faith that things will turn out?

I can dwell on this and get myself way down, but at the same time I know it just takes one patient given up for dead coming through the door with a brand-new healthy and sober life to restore my faith. It's a miracle I witness over and over. In reality, it has very little to do with me. That change takes place entirely inside the person, and I have no idea why. I've heard it attributed to God. That could be right.

Nevertheless, my trip back east leaves me feeling weird, unsettled. The whole time I struggle with difficult emotions: a nagging sense of having been betrayed by the system for not working, by Amber for not getting better, and by myself for not making everything better. The time doesn't pass quickly enough. I can't wait to get back home, and I'm glad when the plane touches down.

Even back at work, I'm thrown slightly off-step by Amber's absence. Until midday, I'm nagged by a sense of unfinished business. No one else is, though. Alexi, the only other staffer who had strong feelings for Amber, doesn't even mention her. We discuss New York, a city she loves, and then the usual routine overtakes us. We have twenty additional patients in beds, all deserving—and needing—the same attention and concern I gave Amber. Not to mention the others who come in daily as outpatients.

What's the old saying? The camel shits and the caravan moves on. That's life in a hospital.

What's life, after all, but a series of problems? And your life is defined by how you handle them.

Over the next three weeks I have plenty to handle. On the positive side, Linsey continues to make progress. One day I see her on the patio, drawing in a tablet. She's quite good; her training as a graphic artist is evident. We get into a fun discussion about art, and trade stories about favorite museums and paintings. She prefers the Impressionists, especially Renoir's *The Boating Party,* which she'd seen years earlier in San Francisco. My choice? Michelangelo's masterwork on the ceiling of the Sistine Chapel.

After that I kept an eye on her. I knew she was working on her second step—*come to believe that a power greater than ourselves can restore us to sanity*—and asking about others. We'd love to see patients get through the third step—*make a decision to turn our will and our lives over to God as we understand him*—but very few have the resources to cover the weeks of hospitalization that can take. The fourth and fifth steps—*a searching and fearless moral inventory of ourselves, and admitting to God, to ourselves, and to another human being the exact nature of our wrongs*—are so intense that some sponsors won't allow their sponsees to begin work on them until they've been sober for six months. Until then they're too fragile, still affected by the biology of their condition. We actually prefer that patients get right to it, as long as they take the time they need to get there.

Linsey's doing just fine. From our brief chats and conversations with other staffers, I know she's trying to deal honestly. One day, as I'm about to leave, she tells me to wait a minute; she has something to show me. She pulls an envelope from the top drawer of her nightstand. The letter, which she carefully unfolds, is from her grandfather in Ohio. She holds up the second page of the letter, and I see a beautiful drawing of a sunflower.

"He said he drew it for both of us," she says.

"It's beautiful," I say.

While admiring the drawing, I see her watching me. When I turn my attention back to her, she maintains contact. That's good. That's what we want.

Why does she seem to get it and Amber didn't? Both arrived in nearly the same condition. Both suffered terrible abuse in childhood. We treated both similarly. So what's the difference?

A few days later, though, I hear that Linsey's leaving. A red flare goes up. What's going on?

Linsey's mother has arranged for her to transfer into a treatment center in Florida that specializes in borderline personality disorders. This is the first I've heard of such a plan. I'm worried that the mother's efforts to inject herself into the process are a subtle way of undermining our work. This sort of thing happens all the time. When a patient starts making progress, their significant others get anxious about the changes. They're used to playing an important role in their loved one's life, and they fear losing that role. Finley and I have a conversation with Linsey's mother. She denies feeling scared or losing control. In fact, she lectures us about being intrusive.

"I'm her mother," she says emphatically. "I only have her interests in mind."

"What about participating in some therapy yourself?" suggests Finley. "If you join in the process, it could be very helpful."

"Excuse me," she says angrily. "I've been involved in the so-called process since she was born."

In the end, we take her blows and lose the patient. Linsey seems to handle it with only minimal anxiety. Honestly, we expected more as she prepared for the discharge and transfer. I catch up with her as she's packing her clothes in an expensive leather duffle bag. She seems somewhat detached and robotic. She explains that her mother has a second home in Florida, along with a sugar daddy and a few relatives there. Some of them are even tolerable, she admits with a smile. She makes a point of showing me that she's taking her steps workbook and says she'll continue listening to *Loveline* from her new home, as she has since she was a teenager. She's actually telling me she wants to keep up the attachment we'd established. Another good sign.

Later that day, after she's been discharged, Alexi hands me an envelope that she says Linsey left for me. I open it up, and find inside her grandfather's drawing of a sunflower. Across the bottom of the stem she wrote, "ThanX." I tack it on the bulletin board in the nursing station as a reminder.

It doesn't hurt to have one, the way things go in the few days that follow. Alexi has begun to suspect two patients of using. Max and Russell started out as roommates, but we split them up as soon as they started to ignore curfews and other little rules. The guys are in their early twenties: Max is a white guy from the dot-com world, and Russell is a black music industry talent scout. Both are opiate addicts. We've had them six days, long enough for them to emerge from the misery of withdrawal and reveal themselves as frustrated, craving, desperate, and full of self-will.

"What worries you?" I ask Alexi.

"They've missed a few groups," she says. "They've had excuses, but

I see the pattern. All of a sudden, like the past two days, neither is participating."

"Urine tests?"

"Both have come back clean the past two days."

Patients sneak drugs and get high during treatment all the time. We don't tolerate it when it we know it's going on, but it happens behind our backs from time to time when they're out of our immediate supervision. Their friends bring stuff in, or they score in the field behind the unit. Desperate people do desperate things. The range of human cleverness and deceit is always impressive. Patients stash drugs in stuffed animals and pillows. There's a huge black market for clean pee. Family members often smuggle in drugs. One patient's husband brought in Oxycontin because he couldn't tolerate her discomfort, which shows the power of the disease over the entire family.

Max and Russell are now marked men. Once Alexi plants the seed, I watch them with a wariness that frequently makes the unit seem smaller than it is. Our paths start to cross more than ever. I ask how they're doing, and they make chitchat. It's all pleasant, but everyone can feel the buildup to something bad.

One night after dinner, as shifts change, a night nurse spots two women she knows from the main psychiatric hospital as they go into Max's room. After Russell follows them in, she calls me on my cell phone while I'm driving to dinner before doing *Loveline*. I instruct her to get the girls out—she calls back later to say she's done so—and the next day Alexi and I speak to the guys separately.

Both of them tell a similar story about the girls coming to their room to continue their AA meeting.

"Right," I say to Alexi.

She laughs. "They're so *devoted*."

We confront them again. "Are you using?" I ask Russell.

"No," he says.

"Is Max?"

"No."

"We have reason to believe there's some drug use on the unit," I say, hoping either to lead him into a confession or simply to scare him. "I want to give both of you a chance to be honest. You know that your treatment contract, which you signed on admission, stipulates immediate discharge for offering drugs to another patient. Relapse can be part of recovery. If you slipped there will be consequences, but you won't be discharged. We want to help you. But we will not tolerate anyone infecting other patients."

"I'm not using," he says. "If you think it's going on, it's someone else. It ain't me."

I'm silent, as is Russell, who looks me straight in the eye with total sincerity. He might even believe it, but my gut tells me he's lying.

Alexi has a similar experience.

Fine. We have no choice but to take their word, and wait to see if something turns up. If they're using, we'll know soon enough.

Later that night, at the radio station, Adam raises an interesting point after a sixteen-year-old girl calls and starts talking about an experience when she was "partying" too much. When did the word *party* evolve from a social celebration, he wonders, to a euphemism for getting fucked up? The phrase "hook up" has recently undergone a similar change. Once it meant to meet a friend; now it refers to indiscriminate, drunken, quickie sex.

"So I was partying too much," the caller continues. "My boyfriend passed out in the living room, leaving me with two so-called friends."

"Why are we so-calling them that?" asks Adam.

"They passed around the bong some more times," she says.

"And you were with them?" I ask.

"Yes. And then one of the guys took me upstairs. I passed out on the bed, and I think he raped me."

"You think he raped you?" I say.

"I sort of remember waking up with him on top of me," she says.

"Did you call for help?" I ask.

"I couldn't. He was so big he scared me."

"Did you tell anyone about this?" I continue.

"No. I didn't want my boyfriend to find out."

She was too comfortable in the role of victim. She was playing the role too well. People don't typically freeze so readily in the face of threat, unless something else has happened earlier in life to set this up. There had to be more.

"Had you ever been raped before?"

"No," she says hesitantly, and then adds, "Well, when I was fourteen I had a boyfriend who did something to me. He was nineteen."

"Listen, this may sound odd, but you seem very comfortable with this stuff that's been happening to you—too comfortable," I say. "Somebody must have done something to you before that. Were you ever sexually abused by someone? Did your parents ever abuse you in some way?"

"My family's great," she says. "I see my dad at least once a month. We have a good relationship now."

"What do you mean now?"

"He left when I was about eleven and we didn't get along so good."

"Did he ever beat you?"

"No."

"He never hit you?"

"Sure, when I was bad I would get whooped. But you know, like everyone, it was just discipline for being bad. I deserved it. No biggie."

There it is. Dad would beat her for her own good. Not only did she feel she'd deserved to be hit, she was cool with it. No biggie. She had just described what human beings do when they have been victimized. First they deal with the overwhelming threat by immediately believing it's something they've caused. I'm wicked and I deserve this. At least that's not as threatening as the reality of their safety being threatened by someone they rely upon for nurturance. Then they learn to detach. In their own minds, it's as if they've ceased to exist—the ultimate disconnect.

"So we never, uh, got to your question," I say. "What'd you want to ask?"

"I missed my period and I don't know what to do."

"You screwball," says Adam.

I take a sip of coffee and tell her.

A few days later, Alexi decides to ruin the afternoon. Not purposely. She's going through the previous night's drug tests, and reads that neither Max nor Russell provided urine specimens within the sixty-minute time period we allow. That's bullshit. It would seem to confirm our suspicions. Then something occurs to me: Max's withdrawal has been too easy.

"I bet he's been chipping," I say. Alexi goes to hunt him down. I'll talk to Russell later. We never confront two patients together; each conversation is confidential and we don't share the information with either individual.

Max acts as if he's surprised I would even want to speak to him. His body language tells a different story.

"You failed to give a urine specimen yesterday in the time period you agreed on in the treatment contract," I say.

"But—"

"We consider that a positive," I continue.

"They didn't tell me I only had sixty minutes," says Max. "I'd just gone and—"

"As I said, it's in your treatment contract. You've been doing it for a week. You should know. I believe you *do* know. What I'd like is for you to tell me the truth."

He doesn't; neither does Russell when I talk with him next. They both deny everything. Russell's much smarter than Max, making me think they may have bonded more out of a desire to use than mutual respect. Russell changes the subject; curious to learn more about him,

I decide to see where he takes the conversation. Very often you get the information you want through a path you didn't see at the start.

"It's not that I'm against returning to the hood in theory," he says. "But I don't have to worry about gangs or gunshots where I live now."

I sympathize. Listening to Russell talk about his family—a cousin who was killed outside a high school, an uncle in prison, his father abandoning him and his two sisters when they were small—and his friends, only a few of whom made it into college, I feel more than just his pain and suffering. If abuse, neglect, and abandonment were viruses, we'd be battling an epidemic so large the country would be engaged in a national emergency. It's in the inner cities, the suburbs . . . it's everywhere.

For some reason, Russell suddenly decides to confess. Something makes him tell the truth.

"Max found some heroin in one of his socks a few days ago," he says, looking away as soon as he finishes.

"Have you used lately?"

He nods.

"When?"

"We—I mean I—both of us chipped a couple times yesterday. I wanted to say no, but I couldn't. It was like I didn't have any control."

"You don't."

"I want to get better. I don't want to be one of those guys who run out of chances. That's why I'm here. I need help."

"Then follow our directions," I say. "We know what we're doing. We've treated hundreds like you. We know what it takes."

We look at each other in silence. I can see his desperation. That's not necessarily a bad thing. I warn him that he might be experiencing withdrawal again. He'll also need to sign another treatment contract, which will include a provision that he'll agree to write about and discuss his relapse in group.

"I don't want any confusion," I say.

"There won't be," he promises.

"If there's any deviation from the contract, even the slightest, you'll be escorted off the grounds immediately."

My next discussion with Max is different. I don't have to reveal what I know. He is aware that information has been passed. This is a bed he made himself, and I wonder how much he will allow himself to get in it. Partway, it turns out. He admits to using, even to getting high earlier that morning, but I can still see his face is a puzzle. He is continuing to maneuver, trying to find a way out. No one is comfortable in these situations. At the same time, they can be an opportunity for a patient to capitulate to treatment at last.

But Max isn't there yet. He says, "I want help," and it's true. Yet I don't see the calm and resignation that come over a patient who means it. Max is continuing to shuck and jive. That tells me it's not over.

"What's going to happen?" he wants to know.

"First, I need to know if you were bringing drugs into the unit."

"No," he says. "Except for what I found in my sock."

"What about the heroin you did this morning?"

"I had a friend come visit. He had some shit. When he offered, I said okay. I couldn't resist. Neither could Russell."

I'm not clear on the biggest issue: whether or not Max gave drugs to anyone. If he did, the punishment is immediate dismissal, no questions asked. He'd be treated like an infecting agent. But I don't know for sure. An addict isn't expected to be able to resist drugs. Max responds like a typical sociopath, trying to make me feel great. He compliments the program and says how much he's getting out of it. He praises me. He seems genuinely sorry. He's suddenly a real people pleaser.

I wish I knew more. Because I don't, I say, "I'm going to give you another chance. The same as Russell."

I believe it's only a matter of time before he screws up and makes the decision for me.

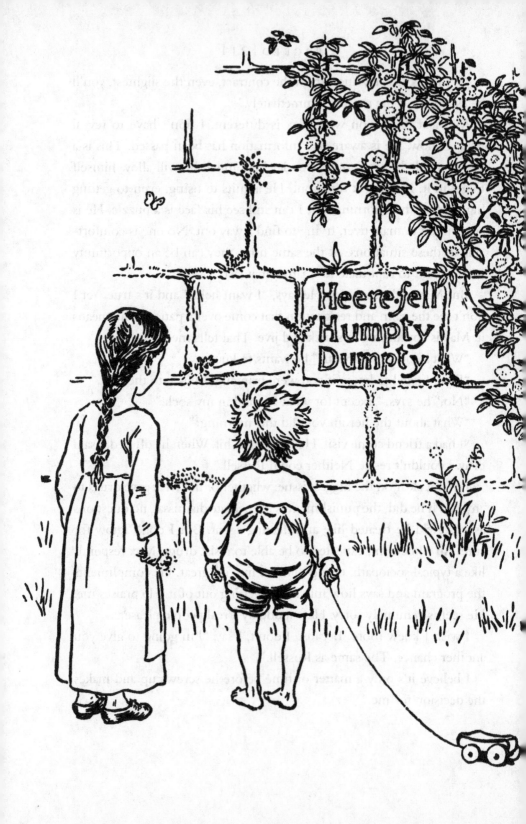

Heere∙fell
Humpty
Dumpty

Twenty-One

THE WAIT ISN'T long. A few days later, Max is caught by the night shift on the corner in front of the hospital doing what we had suspected. I get the news from Alexi the next morning. According to her, Max had convinced the night nursing supervisor to get his wallet out of the safe. He had broken unit restrictions by going outside. There was no doubt why he needed his money. Unable to get me on the phone, the staff contacted Finley, who gave the go-ahead to discharge Max on the spot.

"He was picked up by a friend," Alexi says, putting away his file.

"He wasn't ready," I say. "Too bad. How's his pal?"

"Russell is hanging in," she says.

This will be hard on him. He'll have a lot of mixed feelings, and fear, and he'll have to rely on his peers to help him process Max's sudden departure.

Toward the end of the day Alexi comes into the nursing station from her rounds of the unit. She can't hide her frustration.

"What is it?" I ask.

"You know what I want?" she asks, slapping her palm on the counter.

"What?"

"A good old-fashioned alcoholic," she says.

"Where's our friend Mark Mitchell when you want him?"

But our next patient is transferred from the psych unit. Earle, in his thirties and dressed in a white T-shirt and baggy black pants, is a crack cocaine addict who's out of his mind despite the brief stay in the locked ward. He is sped up, manic, like an airplane bucking out of control. Everything from his movements to his speech is tangential and wild. He keeps insisting to the staff that he and I are friends from childhood. In fact, he even mentions some guys I had known since fourth grade.

I have no idea how he knew those names, not to this day. I had never seen him in my life.

I put Earle on Depakote and Seroquel to calm his mania, and about five days later he finally starts to land. A few days after that we get him to do a first step—and it overflows with atrocities. He says his mother was a heroin addict, and in a monotone voice frightening for its lack of feeling he describes how he came home every day from school wondering if he'd find her alive or dead. Once or twice a month, he would see a fire engine or an ambulance out in front of his house as he walked home from school.

"It got to the point where I changed my pace as I went inside," he tells me one day. "I'd slow it way down. I didn't want to feel a thing. I just asked, 'Is she dead?'"

He saw them cart his mother off while she was frothing at the mouth and covered in shit and pee.

"How old were you?" I ask.

"Eight."

When his mother wasn't incapacitated, she was abusive. She opened their home up to drug addicts willing to trade heroin for a place to crash. He can't remember who did it—it could've been his mother—

but someone gave him pot when he was ten. Around the same time he discovered beer. Both made him feel better. He quickly graduated to harder drugs. As much as he thought he was handling his painful life, he was extremely disconnected. He just grew more addicted.

"How'd you get by?" I ask.

"I ate my Cheerios," he says. "That's all I did. That's all I liked. That bowl of Cheerios."

I find myself drawn to Earle for the wrong reasons. I seek him out for snatches of conversation so that I can look into his eyes.

He also tells me that if need be, he could kill another human being and go back to eating his cereal without a second thought. How could someone get to that point? Think about it. After experiencing one atrocity on top of another, he could no longer trust anyone, no longer connect with anyone; as a result, he could no longer have any of the interactive experiences that would allow him to relate to others, to measure himself against the rest of us.

Why is he able to talk about killing this way, without any hesitation or remorse? Because other people really don't exist to him. One of the higher and later levels of human development is the capacity for empathy. He needs to use other people to survive, but he's a million miles away from recognizing that.

"Why is he here?" asks Pat, one of the counselors, in the team meeting.

"Because of a fuckup, really," says Finley. "He was taken to County Jail, somehow transferred to the hospital, and they shuttled him here."

"He's lucky, in a way," says Pat.

"Drew, how long do you give him?" asks Finley.

"Best case, I'm afraid he's dead in six months to a year," I say. "I can see his pain. I can feel it. I'm not sure he can feel it as much as I can."

"He's completely dissociated when he talks about his life," says Finley. "When he talks about his life, he sounds like he's a narrating a film."

"Only less involved," adds Alexi.

"I think that's how he's been able to survive," says Finley. "He's the modern-day version of Ellison's *Invisible Man*."

"I see someone like this kid and I get angry," I say. "A part of me wants to know why the world can't come to grips with this disease and the causes. Another part of me is grateful to be treating him. Addicts are strong people. They are serious survivors. If you think about it, the whole nature of addiction is about survival in the face of horrible circumstances. It's unusual for an addict not to have some internal resource he can call upon, no matter how horrible the trauma. Apparently Earle's mother was somewhat available to him until she got too strung out, when he was seven or eight. Some of the newer research suggests that a stable attachment in infancy may be enough for someone like this to call upon to rebuild."

"I don't know," Finley says, shaking his head. "Abandonment, chaos, years of opiates. That's a powerful combination to overcome."

But never underestimate the resiliency of the human spirit. I glimpse Earle's inner resources one day following a group. He stops me in the hall and tells me he wants to get better. I have another appointment, but decide this is more important than being on time. I have never sensed anything like this in Earle. I ask some questions, and I get the impression that his mania has settled down. When he first arrived, that's what we had been treating. As he felt better, he began trusting us. He doesn't have family, or a job, or anything else he can look forward to—other than feeling better.

"So what do you want to do?" I ask.

"I want to get the new Radiohead CD," he says.

"No," I say, smiling. "I mean with your life. What do you want to do? What's next for you?"

"I don't know," he shrugs. "You tell me."

Without plans or a place to go, he is asking for guidance. This sounds like a small matter, but it's nothing short of miraculous to me, if he means it. If he's willing to turn to others—and, moreover, others in authority—for solutions. He's lived a life completely without hope of anything but getting through the moment without pain, and suddenly he's been asked something new—he's taken notice of the future. There's no resistance coming off him; he seems to be accepting that his way wasn't working. He seems open to an alternative.

About two weeks later, Earle has completed his behavioral goal: He's gotten a sponsor, completed his first step, and with help drawn up a discharge plan: calling Sober Living, setting up an interview and a move-in date, and creating a schedule of attending groups at the unit as an outpatient.

"You have to be responsible for your own disease and recovery," I explain.

Earle nods and scratches his head. I pat his back. It's not that complicated. It starts with a phone call. Then I leave him to do his thing with the Sober Living intake coordinator. I don't have any idea whether Earle is simply doing what we tell him to, or actually drawing upon an instinct to survive and just looking for a place to crash. What would possibly keep him from using again?

If our roles were reversed, could I make it? I'd like to think I have that strength in reserve. But who the hell knows? I don't know if I could've made it as far as Earle has.

My last interaction with Earle is when I write his discharge order. I shake his hand, wish him good luck, and watch him walk through the doors. He drags a large army surplus canvas bag of used clothes some of the staff rounded up for him. The plan is to see him at eight the next morning for group. He nods affirmatively. A van takes him to Bishop Gooden, a Sober Living facility about ten minutes away.

I give him the thumbs-up sign through the glass door just as Finley passes on his way to his office. I catch up with my colleague a moment later.

"How can you be so matter-of-fact about something like that?" I ask.

"I don't give him a chance," he says. "It's a miracle he's out on the streets and not in jail where guys like him usually end up. How'd that happen anyway?"

"He called and set up the interview yesterday." I shrug. "Whatever we say, he does."

"Maybe he doesn't have any other options."

"I don't think he does. But you know as well as I if these guys haven't capitulated, they'll find ways to keep using."

Sure enough, Earle shows up the next morning at eight. He pedals up on a used mountain bike. Someone at Bishop Gooden had given it to him for transportation. Huffing and sweaty from the long ride, he parks it inside the hall, not even asking if it's okay. I suppose it is. As far as I know, no one's ever ridden up on a bike. Inside, he takes a long breath, gives me a parting nod, and then we walk off in separate directions to do our work.

The same thing happens the next day. And the next. It keeps happening. For reasons I can't explain, he continues to ride to the hospital, always on his bike, and always on time. We don't always cross paths, but I see his bike parked in the entry or I hear about him, and it fills me with encouragement, the type of feeling that fuels hope. We chase so many people out the door, reminding them of their commitment, begging them to return. We don't even have to ask Earle, who just seems to get it.

But then one day he doesn't show up. He comes the next day without explaining his absence. Then he misses the next few. Finally, he stops altogether. He also leaves Sober Living. When we follow up, they tell us that he followed a girl to another facility. Or so they said. Neither left their name.

"I feel betrayed," I tell Finley and Alexi.

"Personally?" he asks.

"No, not personally," I say. "It's a professional failure. First it's Amber. Now him."

"How long have you been doing this?" asks Alexi. "You know how many people don't get the first time."

"Or the second or third," adds Finley.

"Maybe I'm having a crisis of faith," I say. "I don't want to hear this."

"It's the truth, though," he argues. "You can't question Earle. You can't change him, either. What do we tell our patients? They have to take responsibility for their disease and their recovery. If he's going to change—which would be a miracle—it's going to have to come from inside him. I think you're putting too much of yourself into this."

"Maybe I'm not putting *enough* of myself in," I say, raising my eyebrows.

"No," he says. "You're doing as much as the system allows."

"You know what?" I extend my arms in a broad gesture. "I haven't said this since college. But fuck the system."

"I don't know," says Alexi. "The system brought us Earle. The system probably saved his life."

"The system also kicked Amber out. So fuck the system."

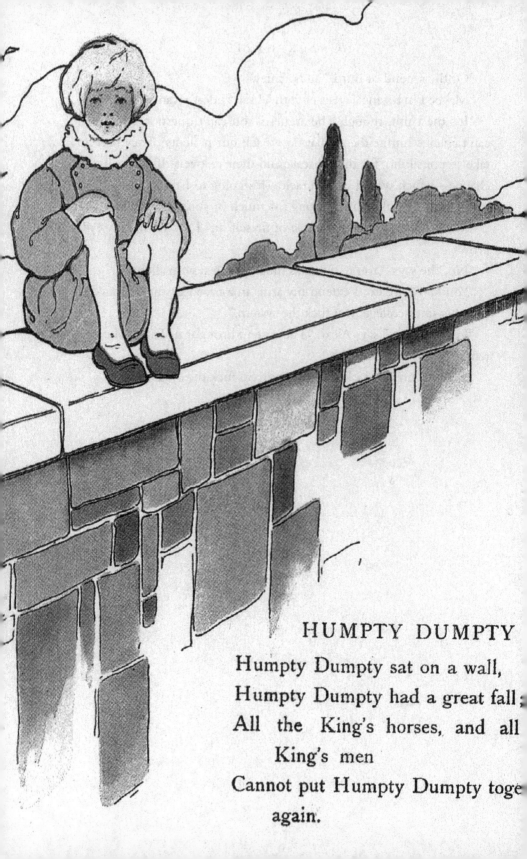

HUMPTY DUMPTY

Humpty Dumpty sat on a wall,
Humpty Dumpty had a great fall;
All the King's horses, and all
  King's men
Cannot put Humpty Dumpty toge
  again.

Twenty-Two

ON THE DAY Amber returns to the unit, I'm treating what Alexi would describe as an old-fashioned alcoholic. Esther, in her mid-sixties, came in during the night. Her daughter brought her. When I enter her room, she's seated on the bed, and she couldn't look thinner or more frail. In her heyday she could never have been more than slight, but now she has no muscle or soft tissue. She's skin and bones covered in a faded orange housedress. I notice she has beautiful coral earrings, though; a hint of life in the past. One of Pasadena's finest.

I pull up a chair and sit down and glance at the few notes on her chart: *Passed out in her apartment. Lives in SQUALOR. Daughter thought she was dead. Smoker. Bad cough. Probably emphysema.* When I take another closer look at Esther, I see she's bruised and banged from falls and accidents, like an old doll. She's also trembling.

"I understand you've been drinking," I say.

"My family would have you believe that," she replies in a weak but coarse and defiant voice.

"Those bruises on your arms—have you fallen recently?"

"A couple times," she says. "It's nothing." She turns toward the window, purses her lips, and gently blows air. "You people won't let me smoke in here."

As if on cue, she rips a big wet cough. I place a hand on her shoulder to steady her.

"I'm fine," she says.

"Those cigarettes need to go, too," I say.

She dismisses me with a simple wave of her fragile hand. For a moment, I can picture her fifty years earlier, a spry young woman at a cocktail party holding a martini glass and a cigarette. The early 1950s. A whole generation of women like her defined themselves by their freedom to smoke and drink. The next generation would partake of drugs and sex. If a show like *Sex and the City* is any indication, the current generation is defined by a desperate inability to maintain a genuine relationship. I'm reminded of the old Virginia Slims cigarette slogan: *You've come a long way, baby.* But is this progress?

Esther coughs into a tissue that was wadded up in her hand.

"Listen, I don't know what all this is about. I'm fine. My daughter gets a fear about me, and the next thing I know I'm in this jail. I want to go home."

"Do you have any medical problems?" I ask.

"No, I told you. I'm fine."

"Have you been in the hospital anytime recently?"

"I don't remember."

"What about for pneumonia? On your chart, I see it says you were pretty sick about a month ago."

"Everyone got all excited about nothing."

Esther is in denial. She's an old woman who totters through her apartment all day with a drink and a cigarette, and when she runs out of booze she shuffles to the nearby restaurant, stumbling up and down the building's stairwell. This is her life. This is how she defines herself.

She is a self-reliant woman who drinks and smokes, and her social life revolves around people who do the same.

Denial; reality. It doesn't matter. Nothing I saw will change that picture.

It's futile for me to argue with Esther. She won't accept any sense of herself that doesn't meet with her approval. The uninformed wonder how people like her can continue to drink when they see what they're doing to themselves. That's the point. You can show them everything from a toxicology report to their reflection in the mirror to their own distraught relatives, but they don't accept it. You've heard of rose-colored glasses? Hers are the color of booze.

According to what her daughter told the night nurse, Esther's drinking picked up in a serious way after her husband died two years ago.

"Ancient history," says Esther when I raise the issue. "Can I go now?"

"This is not a jail," I say. "You can leave any time you want."

"Then call my daughter," she says, her whole body trembling in withdrawal.

She reminds me of a piece of china about to fall off a shelf. She would be in a full-on seizure right now if not for the withdrawal medication we gave her. Extending a steadying hand, I coax her to lie back on the bed and explain that I'll be back to examine her in a little bit. Then I slip out of the room for an appointment having to do with administrative business. Hopefully Esther will sleep for a few hours. Letting her go home would be absurd. We will help her immensely even if we only have her a few days by attending to her medical and nutritional needs. Unfortunately, it's not against the law in this country to drink yourself to death.

I spend the next hour on the phone. It's one of those necessary duties of running a unit within a hospital, like pulling over to get gas when you're in a hurry. It's too boring to go into. During the conference call, though, I see a familiar face through the door. It's Amber. She passes by, walking next to Alexi.

I'm shocked.

When I get off the phone, I immediately find Alexi. She confirms it: That was Amber. Though scattered, she came for a meeting.

"For group?" I ask. "She's hours late for any scheduled outpatient groups."

"I tried telling her," she says. "She couldn't follow. I just sat her down in the group that's meeting now."

"Is she high?"

"She shook her head no."

"I'm worried. But at least she's here."

Before checking on Amber, I have to finish examining Esther. Her condition, it turns out, is pretty much what I expect. Her bruises, the falls aside, are due to her alcoholic liver's failure to produce normal amounts of blood-clotting mechanism. Her legs are swollen, perhaps from heart failure or the added pressure put on her heart by the emphysema. Her lungs are barely functional after years of chain smoking. She has no patience for my poking and prodding. After a few minutes, she squirms free and scoots to the back of the bed.

"I'm too old for this," she snaps.

"Esther, you need to stay here for a while," I say. "If you leave, I think there's a high probability you'll die fairly soon. If you stay, you can feel better."

She isn't happy.

"We're going to focus on getting you stronger," I continue. "You obviously haven't been eating too well. We'll get you on a better diet. I'll also be giving you some medications and vitamin shots, because—"

Just then we're interrupted by a crash, loud enough for everyone in the unit to hear. Both Esther and I stop and turn toward the door. I hear voices down the hall. Advising Esther to lie back down and wait for me, I rush outside just in time to see the end of an altercation at the nursing station between a nurse named Kathy and Amber, who's screaming, "Give me my fucking car keys!"

Amber flails at the countertop. Papers and books fly everywhere. A metal chair falls over, making another crash. I grab a phone on the wall next to me and ask the operator to sound a Code White to the Briar Unit. As soon as Amber hears the alarm sounding through the P.A. system, she sprints down the opposite end of the building, toward the patients' rooms. My first stop is Kathy, who's shaken and breathing hard. She says she's okay.

"What was that all about?" I ask.

"Earlier, I smelled alcohol on her breath," she says. "I was sure she'd been drinking, so I asked for her car keys. I didn't want her driving in that condition. I was going to call her husband to come get her if she refused evaluation to come back as an inpatient. But I didn't even get that far."

"And just now?"

"I'd called the admissions staff to come evaluate her. But they were taking a while, like they always do, and the next thing I know she practically breaks down the door."

"Okay. You did everything right. You're okay?"

"I'm fine."

We have to find Amber. Staff have poured into the nursing station in response to the code announcement. In addition to Kathy, Alexi, and myself, there are six people, all practiced in these sort of events. They happen almost daily throughout the hospital, particularly on the adolescent and locked psych units. Believe it or not, they don't happen as dramatically or as frequently on our unit.

I send two guys outside to look around back in case she's already out the door, and I lead the others down the hall. Kathy thinks she was heading toward her old room. Glancing past the open doors of other rooms as we hurry down the hall, my head fills with the same nagging concerns I had before she was discharged. I'm already jumping to dark conclusions. Then we get to 421. The door is open. The room is empty and tidy. The bed is neat. No signs of anything.

"What about the bathroom?" asks Sean, one of the orderlies. "I smell something burning in there."

The door is shut.

"Yeah, try it," I say.

Sean knocks. Because of Patient's Rights, we can't just burst into a room even when there's a potential danger. After the second quick knock, we hear the sound of breaking glass. It's followed by a thud. He immediately tries the door, but something on the other side prevents it from opening more than a crack. That's enough for us to see Amber lying on the floor, wedged between the door and the toilet. Sean pushes harder, and the door opens.

The first thing I see is a crack pipe on the floor, which I kick to the side. We pick up Amber and quickly carry her to the bed. I bark instructions: "Call a Code Blue. Get a crash cart." I look down at Amber. Her eyes appear to be fixed on a point three feet above her head. They're gray and detached. She swallows once and it's followed by a loud, snapping sound, a shudder deep inside her chest, and a guttural moan. Suddenly I can't get a pulse.

"Get an IV going in that arm," I snap. "Bring me the defibrillator and charge it up to a hundred joules. Set it for Cardioversion."

Nothing happens. I look up at the waiting crew. "Jesus, where's the crash cart?"

Can't waste time. I drop my fist against her chest, hoping to jump-start her heart. I press on her carotid artery. Nothing. I start mouth to mouth.

"Sean, start chest compressions," I say between breaths.

Finally, the cart arrives. According to the monitor her heart rate has risen to 240, with wide complexes. I have Kathy get the EKG pads ready. Someone else gets the Amboo bag and starts running O^2. One part of my brain operates on automatic, while the other is pissed off at the insurance company that forced her out and prevented me from doing the tests my instinct and training told me were necessary. Damn. How can we live with a system where people who don't give a shit make medical decisions?

None of the emergency procedures are working on Amber. Not more adenosine. Not the paddles. Not CPR. Not epinephrine.

She's lying perfectly still, now only a body without life.

Shit. Think. . . .

"Give her another amp of Narcan," I say. "Charge the paddles again. Three hundred joules."

I hold the paddles to her chest.

Clear.

Boom!

Amber's body jumps off the bed as the electricity is delivered; no change. Just as I consider what, if any, last-ditch options are available, the paramedics arrive and take over. Information floods out of me. Amber was probably smoking crack in the bathroom, I tell them. She probably had a flial mitrial valve. I think she had a massive MI, and must have ruptured her ventricle or some other total catastrophe. More . . .

The paramedic nods coolly, never looking up from his clipboard.

They resume CPR, but each squeeze of the respirator bag sprays vomit in every direction. All of us turn away, not from disgust as much as defeat. It is never easy watching someone die. The little room is silent and still and suddenly very claustrophobic. Alexi stands in the doorway. Feeling sick, I hurry past her and into the bathroom. I barely make it to the sink.

I'm there for a while, cleaning up my mess and crying. Finally, sometime later, there's a knock on the bathroom door. It's Alexi.

"Drew, are you all right?" she asks.

"Yeah," I say, lying.

"I couldn't reach Amber's husband," she says. "But her mother's on the phone."

I splash some cold water on my face, take a deep breath, and say, "All right, just a minute."

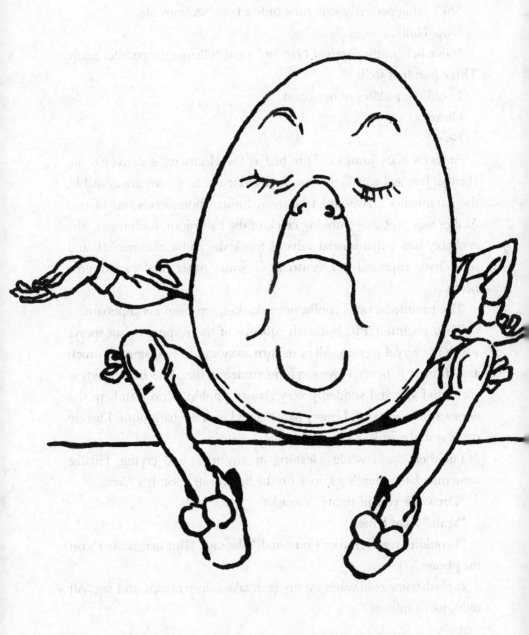

Twenty-Three

FOR THE NEXT two days, I am useless. I stay home from the hospital and let the fact sink in, let it fester: I've lost a patient.

I know exactly what to do for someone else who's suffering. But the magic escapes me as it applies to myself in this hazy time. My wife and children sense the struggle and leave me alone. Several times, when she can no longer stand the sight of me lost in our own home, Susan asks what's wrong.

"Nothing's wrong," I say, and both of us know I'm lying.

I wallow in it. The children come in and out of the room and I don't hear them. I can't sit still in front of the television. I don't want to go for a walk or out to dinner, and when I do I'm not aware of it. Nothing can penetrate the stone wall of depression around me.

On the second night, Susan can't take it any longer. After dinner, she confronts me in the den. I'm in a chair, holding a book on my lap without reading, when she puts her face right in front of mine.

"What's up?" she demands.

I don't want to talk.

She won't let me get away with it.

"I lost a patient."

She strokes the side of my face with her hand.

"I am consumed by thoughts of failure and futility," I say.

I know everyone has a day at work now and then that they want to forget. For me, a bad day isn't a mistake on a spreadsheet, a case that went the wrong way or a missed sale. I had a patient die. A woman in her prime, who should have enjoyed a long and fruitful life, died. Less than a month earlier, I had told her she didn't have to die. I thought she had a chance. I believed it with everything I had. All I wanted was for her to share that belief.

"You're good at what you do," Susan says. "You did your best. It's not like it would have turned out better if you had done something different, or if someone else had been taking care of her."

How can she say that?

I disagree, silently, but vehemently.

She sees that. "Drew, you can't save everybody."

"It's not about that," I explain. "It goes beyond that. Every day I challenge my patients to get better by trusting the program and connecting to other people. They ask how they're supposed to trust, and I tell them to have faith. They want to know, faith in what? Faith in a higher power, I tell them. Where was that higher power when my patient needed it? Where is it now when *I* need it?"

Susan pauses.

"I don't know," she says. "Either you have to find it . . . or it will find you. Or else you're in for one long bummer."

Later that evening, as the sun is setting, I go for a run in the Arroyo, an ancient river basin that runs through Pasadena. In the cool twilight air, amid the long grass and purple flowers on the canyon's walls, I listen to my feet pound the earth and my heart pound inside my chest. I think about the earth and how it continues despite the plunder of humans, beautiful, nourishing, forgiving. I run to avoid defeat, to prove myself, to show I can. Step by step, I conquer boredom, push beyond pain, accomplish something.

Gradually, as I find my stride along the trail, I fall into a meditative state where I am able to open up and search my soul, questioning everything from my own actions to the inaction of the system. I have so much to go over. My thoughts drift from Amber to the pain of so many of my other patients to my place in their lives. What's my purpose in this drama? What's the point, I wonder.

I can't make much sense of anything, but the run feels good.

By the time I return home, I have worked up a healthy, cathartic, cleansing sweat. Susan asks, "Good run?"

"Yeah, good," I say.

"Feeling better?"

"Maybe. I need to shower."

After cleaning up, I walk in on the kids as they watch television. They are completely absorbed by *The Simpsons;* I am taken away by a phone call—Finley calling to check up on me. It's perfect timing on his part. If he had called a day earlier, I would not have been ready to get into it with him. Even a few hours earlier would have been wrong. But now I am ready to talk. Hearing his voice unlocks the door to the vaulted emotions that have paralyzed me for the past forty-eight hours. After listening to me, he offers another slant on the situation.

"Blame yourself if you want. Feel sorry for yourself if you want," he says. "But why don't you also blame her?"

"You know why? She had no control over the disease. We didn't provide enough help."

"We did what we could," he argues.

"I don't know," I say. "We knew what we needed to do. We needed to nurture a trusting connection and maintain it. We really didn't do that."

"Was there willingness on her part?"

"I believe so. Only a month ago she admitted that she didn't want to die. She was in tears as she said it. It was as if she had a premonition. But that's not the point. The point is that I had gained Amber's trust, but to what end? To suffer one more abandonment and set her up for an even bigger and more tragic collapse?"

"Maybe you're right. But the fact is, sometimes you don't get the breaks. You can't be the hero every time."

He makes his point and then changes the subject to something lighter. The Dodgers are always good for a few minutes of distraction. After hanging up, I am still confused. There is no simple or easy resolution. I read for a few hours and then slide into bed next to my wife. Though she's already sleeping, Susan's leg touches mine, and that feels good.

The next morning it's time to go back to work, something I can feel in my bones. I step back into the morning routine of getting the paper, making coffee and conversation with my wife and kids. All of this is a tremendous source of comfort. Returning to work isn't as smooth. I walk in with a certain amount of dread.

The unit is quieter than normal. Like me, everyone is still dealing with Amber's death. Whenever something like this happens, whether it's someone getting caught with dope or someone dying, there are repercussions. Usually patients get their shit together for a little while. They settle down like a restless population after a public beheading.

"How are things?" I ask Alexi as she brings a fresh cup of coffee to the nursing station.

"It's slow," she says. "I'm bored."

She makes no mention of my two days off. Neither do I. We go on as if nothing has happened.

My first patient is Esther, the older woman I had been examining when the episode with Amber started. Because we were interrupted in midexam, I want to go back and reestablish contact with her. I find her in her room shortly after she has been brought back in a wheelchair after a short stint sitting in the morning sun on the patio. I ask if she knows how many days she has been in the unit.

"Too many," she says.

"You've been here three days," I say.

"You're right."

She is lethargic, thick-tongued, and unstable (hence the wheelchair) from the Librium we have given her to suppress the alcohol withdrawal. For older people with other medical problems, withdrawal is really dicey. They can easily lapse into a potentially fatal state of delirium tremens and quickly slip away.

But Esther, for all her problems, is hanging in there. She is even thinking fairly coherently through the medication.

"I heard what happened to that girl," she says.

"Yeah."

"What's a matter with kids today?"

I shrug. What am I supposed to say? That they're overstimulated, bored, drugged out, and disconnected from each other?

That they're fucked by pop culture?

That they're lost?

I don't have to say anything. Esther can't identify with the kind of turmoil and chaos of young women like Amber. She tells me that women of her generation facing adversity got their shit together. End of story.

"I don't get it," she says. "We drank at lunch. But we didn't get tattooed or stick pins in our tongue or our eyes."

She coughs.

"I don't know what to say," I tell her.

"It's okay if you don't want to talk about it."

"About what?"

"The girl that died."

"I don't know if I do or I don't."

"You did the best you could," she says. "You guys work so hard. I see how you and the others go all around and help everyone."

"Thanks."

"You can't save them all."

"What do you mean?" I ask in a slightly mocking tone.

She taps a finger on her chest as if to say, "Look at me. Here's another one you aren't going to save."

Enough about me. We need to readdress Esther's treatment more than we need to discuss my needs. Glancing at notes on her chart, I see her daughter was here the night before—merely to visit, though, not to participate in family group or any other aspect of treatment. I get it. She just wants Esther fixed. She doesn't want to do anything that would require examining herself.

That's normal among families. All too often family members don't really want the patient well. They want them the way they were before the addiction got out of control. Fundamental emotional change is too scary; it can often require family members to look at their own emotional issues, which can be a major stumbling block.

"How was your daughter?" I ask.

Esther shrugs. "I asked her to take me home. She said no. Then I asked her not to talk while I watched television. She left."

"I can see you're feeling better," I say.

She shrugs again, but it's the truth. Three days of good food, rest, medication, and no drinking have improved her health. Granted, we're letting her smoke outside, so she's happy. She lets me know she could be happier.

"When can I go home?" she asks.

"I don't know," I say.

"Doctor," she says, pointing her trembling hand at me. "What's the point? What are you going to do for me—really?"

"We're going to make you feel better."

"That young one—you might have been able to do something for her. But she's dead. So for me? I'm seventy-two years old. I've got how many years at most—eight? Ten? What's being sober going to do for me?"

Her logic kind of staggers me. A part of me wants to admit she has a point. It's a little like the situation I sometimes face when I argue against withholding morphine from an opiate addict with cancer, though I have found that frequently addicts with a strong connection to sobriety will want to go through as much pain as they can stand without drugs. It's their choice. Esther's giving me the same message. Whether she has two years or ten, she wants to live them with her friend and lover, alcohol.

"Could you be happier sober?" I say. "I honestly think you would. Would you benefit medically? Yes. Would it prolong your life? Probably."

"And your point?"

"You'd have a fuller, more complete life experience."

She brushes aside my argument with a shake of her head and announces that she's going outside to smoke a cigarette. "I would prefer it with a cocktail."

I might as well have tried selling Esther on ginseng tea, or asked to her to reconsider the feng shui of her apartment. We are on different planets.

I step into the hall, realizing that, though Esther has no more use for me, she has in fact caused me to ask a serious question.

What am I really doing here?

What's the point?

I once had a discussion with an aquaintance about mental health. This guy was a brilliant businessman involved in the entertainment industry. We were having dinner at a mutual friend's house, celebrating one of his latest multimillion-dollar deals. At some point he turned his attention to my work. After listening to a few stories about my work with patients, he said he could improve the results I got by developing a "happiness scale."

"You have these troubled individuals who can't really express their suffering or their joy," he said. "But if you created a scale, you would be able to quantify their feelings. Instead of pain, you could be measuring happiness."

"How do you figure out the scale?" I asked. "What's a one? What's a ten?"

He needed only a moment to formulate his spreadsheet logic.

"Well, take me, for instance. I guarantee you that I'm way up on the happiness scale. I have a beautiful wife. Two kids. And I just sold one of my businesses. I couldn't be better."

Without using him as a specific example, I took exception to his theory.

"What the fuck are you trying to say?" he eventually asked, unable to reckon a world where numbers weren't primary.

"I'm saying that I don't think happiness should be the goal."

Esther, I think as I walk from her room, is happy when she has a bottle close by. No one is happier than my heroin addicts when they first get going with their drug of choice. Pot addicts are the same when they're lighting up. In that moment they have found the solution, and everything is okay. You can't find folks who are happier.

I'm aware that I'm pondering this question at a time when I am at a low point of my own, feeling inadequate and unworthy. I am definitely not happy. I'm not walking around with a smile on my face. I am not offering high fives to friends, neighbors, and co-workers, going, "Hey, let's hear it for being happy."

But "happy" is such a ruse. I deal with actors and rock stars and Hollywood executives who have wealth, fame, drugs, sex, great homes, the best tables in the finest restaurants, five-star vacations in exotic locales . . . they have everything—including the misery, pain, and suffering of addiction. Kurt Cobain . . .

(Fill in your own list of celebrity ODs)
1._____
2._____
3._____

They aren't happy people.

If not happiness, then, what?

Better that we start at a more basic level: mental health.

Mental health is defined by one's ability to be fully present and integrated in reality. Of course, that reality may not always be happy. There might be negative experiences. In fact, there will be negative experiences, days that are downright crappy, moments or even years so painful you'll ask why such shit is happening to you. But if you are mentally healthy, you will be able to tolerate such experiences, regulate your emotions. And in the end you will be nourished by something more real than merely "feeling good."

Later that afternoon Alexi and I are due at one of our regular staff meetings across the grounds. As always we take the walk together, enjoying the moments outdoors. The path, snaking across a parklike stretch of grass, is lined with flower-filled gardens. It is empty and serene. We see several squirrels, a lizard, and an array of birds. One patch of grass in the shade is full of enormous black crows.

"What do they know?" I wonder, motioning toward the birds.

"They know where the worms are," Alexi says, laughing.

We move on for several moments in silence, until I catch Alexi looking up at me as we walk. We stop and I ask, "What?"

"Are you okay?" she asks.

I know what she is talking about. I have been absent from work, troubled, distracted, irritable, depressed, quiet, and confused, and she has read me like a menu.

Still, I am not forthcoming. "What do you mean?"

"How are you doing with all of this?"

"I'm okay," I say, surprised to hear those words coming out of my mouth.

"I don't believe it," she says. "No, you can't be. Not without me mothering you a little bit."

I chuckle. We get into a brief discussion about medical responsibility.

"I hope you don't feel mistakes were made," she says. "Or there was something more you could have done."

"The system sucks. That's not our fault. She shouldn't have died. That's the reality. And I'm not sure we couldn't have done things a little different. But"—I sigh—"I'm okay."

"What do you mean you're okay? You seem upset."

"I am upset. It's painful. But I'm dealing. What about you? You loved your little pain in the ass."

"Well, I cried," Alexi says. "I cried that first night. My husband and child wanted to know what was wrong. I told them. We talked about it. I cried some more and then I didn't have to anymore. Now I'm nervous."

"About what?"

"I'm nervous we should be doing more. I'm nervous that if we don't do more someone else will die."

"You know what? Someone else is going to die. Eventually. But our treatments are good. Our program is right. We know what we're doing. We can help people. We have to keep doing the best we can."

We start to walk again, but as I replay my last comment I hear my inner voice say, *Wait a minute. You have to do better than that for Alexi.* Everything I'd just said was uttered on autopilot. Obviously I'm still a little vulnerable, and I was feeling invaded by Alexi's feelings. But Alexi is in this, too, and shifting into neutral that way was no good or fair or helpful for either of us. I need to mark her feelings and listen, acknowledge her concern and pain. I need to connect. So I stop and look straight into her green eyes, and ask her to go on.

After a few moments of conversation, Alexi calms down. To my surprise, I didn't have to rescue her from her feelings. I just had to be there, and she calmed down. My empathy was enough. I felt more secure. This is new to me, a small but significant change in awareness.

I realize we can't save each other. But we can be there for each other. We can be open, empathetic, present.

And I was still there for me.

"How are the kids?" she asks, turning it back on me.

"They're great," I say. "They're playing baseball and ice skating, they're doing well."

We start walking again. We have to get to the meeting. As it is, we're going to be late. I wish I could stay in the moment a little longer, because I sense that it's some kind of breakthrough, a door Amber has opened, a debt I will owe her. A slight breeze picks up. I have a small tear in my eye and a warm spot in my heart. Before entering the administration building, I tell Alexi that I'm grateful for her friendship, for her health, and for her partnership.

She shakes her head. I'm sure she wants to make some crack: "What kind of dope are you on?"

But she doesn't say anything, and we go into the meeting.

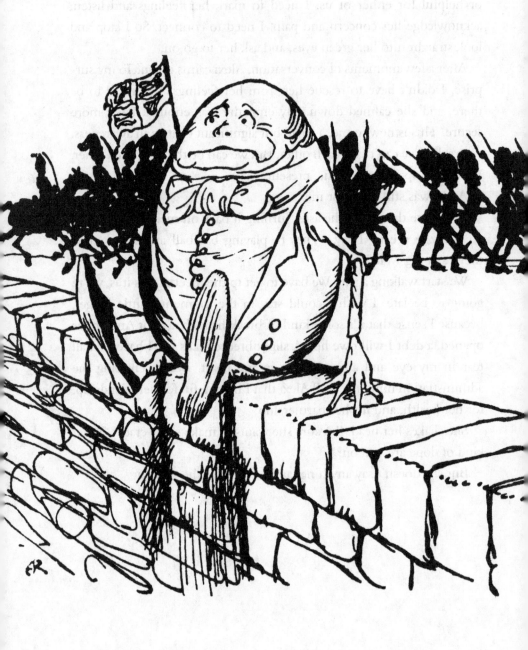

Twenty-Four

IT IS TWO days later, and I am listening to the crackly rattling in Esther's lungs. They sound like metal garbage cans rolling around an alley. Her bruises aren't healing. She's still drowsy from the Librium, and so I cut that back and switch her to Serax, a similar drug that is metabolized differently. It should enable her to wake up, but I can't provide anything that will allow her to tolerate treatment any better.

I can see she is fed up. She shuddered away from me as I tried examining her. She doesn't want to cooperate.

"I'd like you to start attending groups more regularly," I say.

"Oh no, I can't listen to those stories," she says. "There's no one my age, and I'll tell you something. Those young people in there are disgusting. Their language is horrible. You can't imagine the kind of words they use. I can't tolerate that. It makes me too upset. I can't even *say* those words."

"You don't have to," I say. "Just sit there."

"Why? To hear those stories? The things those women talk about. The men are so violent. It's frightening."

I understand. She doesn't identify with any of the other, mostly younger patients. But I really don't know what to do.

I don't have many options. I can't threaten her with a discharge, since that's what she wants. So over the next week I make it a point to try to develop a warm connection with her, and hope she stays long enough for her daughter to take a more active interest in her treatment. At the same time, she emerges from her Librium cocoon and provides enjoyable company, even if it is irascible. Esther wins over a lot of the staff with her no-nonsense talk. She seems to have a comment on almost any subject, especially the younger people.

"I think a lot of the kids you got here just needed a good paddling when they were young," she says.

"A lot of them did get hit," I reply.

"They didn't get hit in the right places," she cracks.

The last time I see Esther, she's talking about politics. She doesn't know much about current events, which is surprising for the amount of television she watches—her set is on 24-7—but "the old lady," as she has lately taken to calling herself, definitely has her opinions. She thought JFK was sexy. His brother Bobby, too. "But not Teddy," she adds. "The rest of those Kennedys are from nothing." She has no liking for Nixon or Ford. "I liked Carter and his mother, Miss Lillian. She was a kick in the ass."

"What'd you think of Reagan?" I ask.

"Handsome."

"How about Clinton?"

"He was a honey."

"Bush?"

"I want to live long enough to see a regime change," she says, borrowing a phrase from the latest war, and showing me she might be more with-it than I suspect.

Esther is much improved from the time she was admitted. No question. Having regular meals, decent sleep, and no booze has made her stronger and healthier. I see potential for a few good years, even if she doesn't. Yet I don't know what to do with her. Then she solves that problem late in the afternoon. It's about four-thirty, and I'm helping Alexi prepare for the next team meeting when I look up from a stack of folders and see Esther teetering down the hall, holding a tiny bag with her belongings, like a little old lady heading toward her train.

In her case, it's a cab.

"I've called a taxi," she says.

I'd wondered if this would happen. It typically does with the more able elderly patients. At a certain point, they reach their limit and go.

I look at Alexi, who has her hand on the stack of files. If she has strong feelings about a patient, she usually shares them. This time she remains silent. I make a few comments to Esther about staying, but they're halfhearted. Both of us know it. I really can't think of anything more to do for this patient, but she has a parting comment that's intended to help me.

"This place isn't for me," she says. "But you keep up the work. You've got to help these kids."

"I will," I say. "Take care of yourself."

Alexi and I make sure Esther gets to the taxi.

"That was interesting," she says after it drives off.

"What was?" I ask.

"Before, you would've fought and threatened her. You wouldn't have given in so easily."

I shrug.

"Maybe I'm changing."

A while later I check on the patient in 419. Brianna is a nineteen-year-old competitive gymnast who came in addicted to speed a few hours before Amber died. She was placed in the room next to Amber's. After Amber died, Brianna freaked out, complaining she'd never been that close to a dead body. She stood in the hallway, warning us she didn't want to see the body, and going on and on about it until someone stepped away from the commotion long enough to say, "Then get in your room."

She has struggled the past three days with boundary issues. She has shown up late to her groups. She has taken over the television set in the lounge, fixating on certain sexy programs that feed her need for a thrill. We have had to curtail that habit. Now, since the previous evening, she has convinced herself that her chronically ill grandfather back east is going to die at any moment, and so she wants out. She's still harping on it when I check on her.

"No one here understands how close we are and how much he means to me," she says.

"Yes, we do," I say. "We also understand what you're feeling, and why, and you need to start showing up in group on time and talking about it."

She turns toward the window, and with one finger delicately parts the drapes a sliver so she can see outside.

"But I could've been that girl who died," she says. "It freaks me out. I can see the same thing happening to me."

"That's right," I say. "That's your disease. She had it, too, and it killed her. It kills lots of people. I don't want that to happen to you."

"It wasn't supposed to happen to her, either," she says. "I mean, this is a hospital, for crying out loud."

"Yes, it's a hospital. People die at hospitals. They also get better—the way you will if you share this, get a sponsor, work on your first step, and get this process going. It's painful. All these feelings you have now are the ones you've been covering up with all this behavior. It's time to feel the feelings."

It's also time to contain Brianna better. We limit her TV, take away her cell phone, and make sure she gets to group on time. Basically we close down all of her escape hatches, hoping she learns to calm down. It doesn't work immediately. For a day and a half, she gets profoundly depressed. She also suffers two panic attacks.

Somehow, though, amid all this drama, Brianna connects with another patient, Azura. In her mid-twenties, Azura looks completely unapproachable. Her arms, neck, and back are totally covered with tattoos. She is pierced on her tongue, nostril, and cheek. She looks like a tribal desperado from a Mad Max movie. The two women couldn't look more different on the outside—and yet Brianna and Azura have soon found a common ground for sharing in a way that makes them see how similar they are on the inside.

Still, I couldn't be more pleased. For Brianna, this is an important step that could be the start of real healing. She is connecting with another person. And vice versa. That's exactly how it happens. It can't happen any other way. If both women are going to make it in recovery, they need to be involved with something other than themselves. A genuine self can only develop in relation to someone else. In the past, people turned to loved ones, neighbors, or religion to heal their problems. That doesn't happen anymore. Nowadays the culture is all about arousal and quick fixes. But they don't work.

The way these two women click has the potential to be different, to be the real thing. I can't predict if it will turn out well for them. It is a long process, much longer than the twenty-eight days (max) that most patients spend in the unit. It is a process that will take the rest of their lives. Yet I hope I am witnessing a vital step in what could be their chance at a new, more fulfilling life. This is how it begins.

Apparently something else is beginning, too. I don't notice it, but Alexi comments on my mood, my reaction.

I take a step back from myself and agree.

"I think hope has returned."

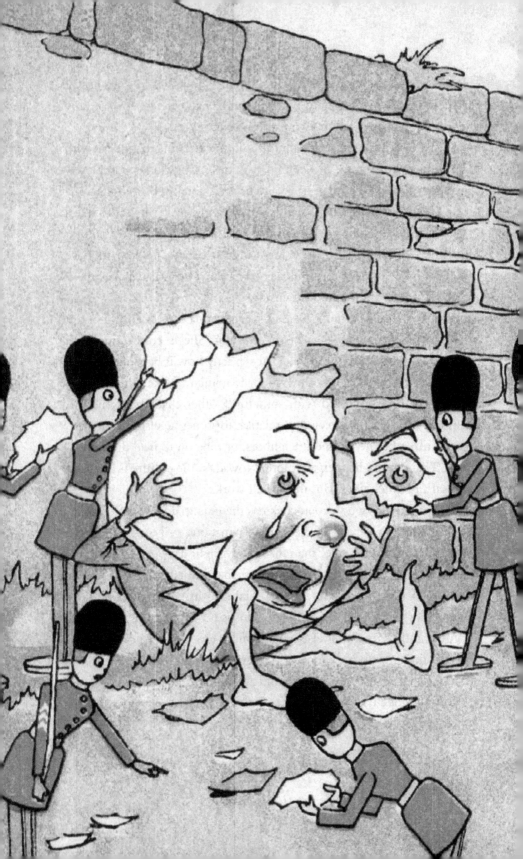

Twenty-Five

IT'S A LOVELY afternoon, several months later, and I step up to the front of the line at the bookstore and watch with pride as the woman behind the register rings up a few new pieces of summer reading for me. It is Hannah, one of my former patients. Working in a small town like Pasadena, I run into my former patients all the time. Hannah is pleased to see me.

"Oh my god, I love this stuff," she says, gesturing to one of the novels I'd picked up. "Have you read him before?"

"Nope—first time."

Hannah looks great. I don't sense the emotional chaos that seemed to accompany her before. She is well groomed and seemingly together.

"I'm so glad to have a job," she says, dropping my receipt in the bag. "You should stop by the café next door on the way out. Everything there is delicious. You can see that by the pounds I've put on."

"You look terrific," I say.

"I'm sober," she beams. "I'm so grateful."

Hannah goes on about the regular work she does with her sponsor. She sounds genuinely pleased. She seems stronger. But what about her daughter? Hannah sighs. That has been tough. Her daughter has been terribly angry with her, but she has started to attend Alateen meetings, which she hopes will help temper those feelings.

"I can't blame her for hating me some," she says. "After all, she has a right to be angry at me."

"You're right," I say. "She's trying to come to terms with her own life, and no one can change her reality. She needs a chance to deal with it. The better you do, the better chance she has."

Before I leave, Hannah leans over the counter. Her fingers tap the glass top.

"Is it kosher for me to ask what's happened to some of the others who were in treatment with me?" she says. "You get so close to some people, and then they disappear. I really hope they're doing okay."

"Who do you want to know about?"

"Well, Wendy. She was a wild one."

"Unfortunately, I don't know what happened to her. After two months in Sober Living, she got into an all-women's program. That's the last I heard."

"What about Linsey?"

"Not good. After two weeks at a facility in Florida, she returned to L.A. One of the counselors ran into her at a meeting. She's been struggling with her sobriety."

"What about that real pretty girl? She was kind of weird. Kind of quiet. I don't remember her name."

"Amber?"

"That's her. What happened to Amber?"

I look across the bookstore, through the window, and onto the street where a woman in running clothes is pushing a baby stroller in the crosswalk. For the next few minutes I provide Hannah with the sad details. She interrupts several times to ask questions, including several having to do with Amber's insurance, and as she talks, she picks at a plate holding tiny sample pieces of blueberry, cranberry, and bran muffins.

"The poor thing," she says, before doing something completely unexpected. She asks, "How are you doing?"

Good question. Several months have gone by, and I have calmed down. Calm might not be a typical reaction to the death of another, but since that tragic incident I have felt calmer. It took a while. I had to live through the emotional mess that followed her death. But as time passed, I acquired a sort of clarity. That, and I became more accepting of my role in the events as they transpired. As I told Hannah, I did everything I could.

Once I was able to figure out what I had gone through, I felt relief. I felt release. I felt open, whole, and calm.

Calm is a new feeling for me. Ever since my episode with the man with the crosses in his eyes, I have spent my entire life focused on the well-being of the people around me, struggling to prevent bad things from happening to them. If I kept them well, everything would turn out all right, and I would be okay. I would ward off the sense that a catastrophe was always around the corner.

I was a resident the first time I had to confront the fact that reality didn't always cooperate. It was in 1982, and I was on call at County General. It was past midnight, well past, and the cardiologist on duty asked me to taper a seventy-five-year-old woman patient off life-sustaining pressors—medication that maintained her blood pressure and kept her heart muscles pumping.

I looked at him as he gave the instructions, hoping on one hand that he wouldn't notice the beads of sweat appearing on my forehead, while on the other hand thinking perhaps he would see the question marks in my eyes and explain why now, at this moment, with traffic in the halls at a minimum and beds plentiful, he decided to have *me* end this woman's life simply by turning a knob. But he barely glanced up from his clipboard before walking away.

"Got it," I said.

I had seen the patient before. She was sick beyond repair or hope, after more than a decade of physical decline, and both she and her family had issued clear instructions not to prolong the end if her basic quality of life could not be guaranteed. Wise, sensible, matter-of-fact. The patient and her kin had already come to terms with death.

I had a harder time. I went into her room, where it was just the two of us, along with several machines that were turned off, and a tall IV stand holding several bags of life-sustaining fluids connected by long clear tubes to her thin arms. I don't know if she was conscious, or floating through a more pleasant place in a faraway dreamlike state of mind, but her eyes were open, and I swear to God she was looking directly at me. I stood at the end of her bed, thinking about it all, until I realized I was only spooking myself.

The woman's breathing was weak and mechanical. After summoning my nerve by taking a deep breath myself, I performed the assigned task. I reduced the pressors and watched the reaction in the patient. It was instantaneous. The life drained out of her. Her breathing grew faint, her eyes sank, and her gaze became fixed.

I had an immediate reaction, too. I got scared. *Oh shit, I've just killed this woman.*

Then, as if on impulse, I turned up the medication, and watched the patient come right back, just as she'd been when I walked in the room. For a moment, I felt relieved. I asked myself how the cardiologist could have been so nonchalant in his instructions to me. Then I realized I knew the answer already. She was sick beyond repair, someone who would never have any more than the most tenuous grasp on life as long as she was given these drugs. Was this living?

I reduced the pressors again. But as soon as she began to die, I turned them on again.

Finally, I went back to check with the cardiologist once more. "She needs to be allowed to die," he said.

That was it, then. I went back and watched the patient drift away. It ran counter to every sensibility I had. I thought doctors were supposed to *save* people from dying. But in this case I actually had to help one die. The experience might have made me quit medicine, but instead it made me a better doctor. I discovered that some deaths were good deaths. As I moved on, I found that I focused more and more on the pain and suffering in the lives of my patients. I defined myself by what I could do for others, which was alleviating pain and lessening suffering in my patients. They, in turn, just had to listen to me. And if they didn't? Well, they had to. If I did my job well, other people wouldn't have any other choice except to cooperate with me.

Of course it's unreal to think I should be able to save everyone or that everyone should listen to me or both. How dare I insist all my patients cooperate with my need to rescue? But that's exactly what I did.

As a result, I became so preoccupied with everyone else's needs that I neglected my own. I was like many of my patients, closed off to the emotional nourishment I needed to develop a healthy self, I became unable to regulate my feelings, and so I turned to rescuing other people the same way my patients turn to drugs and alcohol. But my feelings about Amber pressed my face to the mirror. It was my bottom. I had to change.

I did so without being fully aware that the plates of my consciousness were slowly shifting. My healing process began with my run along the Arroyo, then continued with talks with Finley and Alexi and my wife and my patients, people who in their different ways caused me to recognize the fallacy of my omnipotent self-image. But I was not really conscious of the way those talks have percolated in me until I spoke to Hector, a former patient who approached me after one of my weekly medical lectures and asked for a moment in private.

Of course I'm happy to talk with him, and he waits patiently while

I answer questions from a handful of other current and former patients. When I'm done, I suggest we talk while walking back toward the unit, because I have to pick up my daughter at the ice skating rink.

"How old is she?" Hector asks as we fall into step.

"Ten."

"My daughters are ten, too," he says.

That's right. I remember now: Hector has twin girls. The twenty-six-year-old ex-gangbanger is a devoted father. When I first came into his room and asked why he was there, he said, "I don't want my girls to be like me."

Hector had been surrounded by death his whole life; it was a miracle he was alive. The youngest of three boys born and raised in the roughest section of East Los Angeles, he barely knew his parents. His father was sent to prison when he was five, and his mother died of a heroin overdose when he was nine. His two brothers were both gunned down in gang fights. Growing up alone, Hector managed to escape the neighborhood when he somehow lucked into a job as a pharmacy tech.

But his break wasn't totally clean. A heroin user since his teens, he was unable to resist easy access to drugs at the pharmacy. He started with Vicodin. He controlled his habit for a while with periodic blasts of naltrexone, an opiate blocker that shocks the body into a rapid withdrawal. Then he found Dilaudid, and that was that. After his boss discovered him semiconscious in the back room with blood trickling from his forearm vein, he ended up in rehab.

I liked him immediately. His honesty was raw, right out there on the surface. He was motivated. He didn't play games. His employer, a middle-aged man who ran a mom-and-pop pharmacy, stuck by him. Hector reached out to others in group, and found that people responded to him. He seemed to get it. Now, eighteen months later, he was wrestling with a problem that could destroy his sober life.

We stop walking and Hector looks straight into me. I see the anguish in his eyes.

"I keep thinking I'm going to die soon," he says.

This strong young man covered with tattoos is trembling with fear and nerves. I put a hand on his shoulder.

"Like your mother?" I ask.

"Like everyone I know," he says. "I'm no different than her, or my brothers, or all the kids I grew up with. I'm just waiting, man. I can hear the bomb ticking. I can't sleep. I can't concentrate on anything. The feeling never goes away. I don't know how to make it go away. I just keep thinking it's going to happen any moment."

I don't tell him, but I know too well what it's like to think that catastrophe is around the corner. Still, I can't help pushing Hector a little bit: I know he's stronger than this.

"I guess you're already dead then, right?" I say. "You're not worth it. It doesn't matter anyway what you do. It's hopeless, right? So just fuck it."

"Yeah, fuck it. I might as well get high."

"How does it feel to be dead?" I ask.

He bristles with anger and aggression. "What are you talking about?"

"I want to know how that feels. Tell me."

He struggles against the challenge. I see his frustration and fear as he bumps into feelings the human mind loathes.

"How does it feel? It feels fucking *empty,* man." Suddenly Hector is in my face, nose to nose, angry and aggressive. He yells, "Are you really interested in fucked-up feelings, doc?"

I am, but not at this close range. Suddenly the whole outdoors seems too cramped. "Hey, Hector," I say, "you're standing so close I can't make things out clearly. I'm not only getting old, I guess I'm also going blind. Would you mind taking a step back?"

Hector pulls back and smiles. Casting his eyes downward, he shakes his head. My playful response forced him to connect momentarily and see the experience from my perspective. For a moment I truly existed for him as a separate being with my own feelings. I wasn't angry with him for letting out a little aggression toward me. Equally important, I wasn't ashamed for having triggered them. Nor was I inclined to be responsible for soothing him and rescuing him from his feelings.

"Hector, you're not dead," I say, seizing the opportunity to open up his feelings to him a little bit. "That emptiness is something people escape into when they have no other escape. When you were a kid and your dad beat the shit out of you and your mother died, you survived by dying emotionally."

"Yeah."

"Whenever you're scared or anxious, you go there. It doesn't matter if you make a mistake at work, get in an argument with your wife, think about your kids, or feel like you might want to use again. It's anything and everything you can't control. You imagine yourself dying. You see death. It's really emptiness, but it can feel like death."

"Yeah." He nods.

"But it's not real. In fact, it's as unreal as thinking you can control everything and everyone." As I hear my voice, I realize I might as well be talking about myself. Or *to* myself. "You know, real recovery is about accepting powerlessness. It's about accepting that you were traumatized, and while that was intensely, seriously wrong, you survived. Appreciate that. You got a chance. Your life can be okay. You can't be perfect. You can't ever be pain-free. But things can be okay."

"How do I know that?" he asks.

"You work hard, you do what you're supposed to do, and you have faith."

"Faith?"

"Yes, have a little faith. It's the thinnest strand and it holds all of us together. You have to trust me and have a little faith. Eventually, over time—I can't say when—you'll have a sense that something profound has happened. Everything will be the same, and yet something will be different."

"What's that?" he asks.

"You won't feel dead."

"How will I feel?"

Good question. I think for a moment.

"You will feel whole."

I don't expect Hector to understand at this stage. I barely do myself. But he walks back to the unit. I get in my car. And I think both of us feel better.

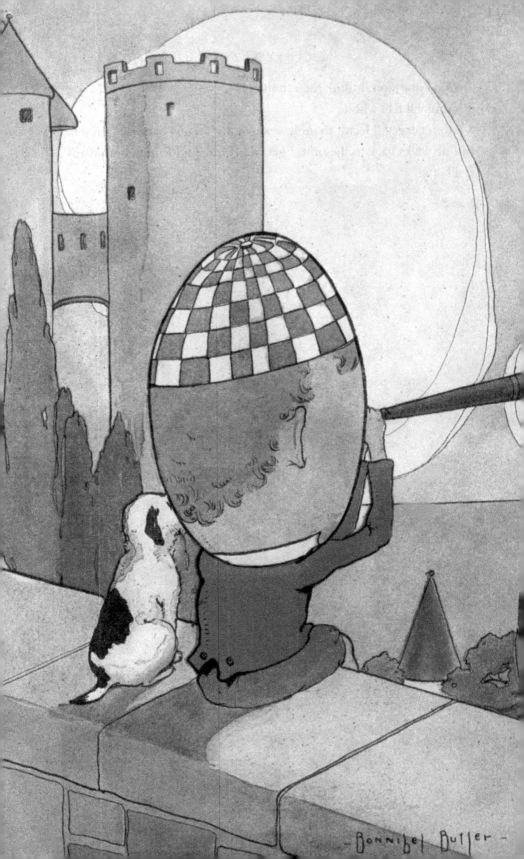

Twenty-Six

THE NEXT DAY is Saturday, and I stop at the unit before meeting my wife and kids at a birthday party at the park. The sky is a dull gray blanket of clouds bringing cool air from the ocean. I cross paths with Finley walking toward his office. He says something about the two of us working weekends, as if we were kids out of graduate school. I smile, though it doesn't feel like work; it's just what I do.

"I sent you a couple of adolescents who called my office looking for a therapist," I tell him.

"I know," he says. "I talked to one, saw the other. The moms are nuts. It's never just the kids. Both dad are alcoholics, completely checked out of their lives. The moms are compensating by hyper-achieving and acting out their needs through the kids. Don't worry, though. I'll get them."

"Great," I tell him. "See ya later."

I cut through the patio behind the unit, interrupting two squirrels and a crow picking over the remainder of a breakfast tray left out on a table among the ashtrays.

"Sorry," I say to the animals.

Inside, I see Alexi at the nursing station. I am surprised. She is supposed to be off. She says the same about me, and we laugh. She explains that Jane, her weekend counterpart, came down with the flu. She wants to know why I'm standing in front of her when she knows I am supposed to be at one of my kids' events.

"I got a call last night that Debra came back," I say. "I wanted to check on her."

Debra is the wisecracking junior TV executive who was in a few months ago for a Vicodin and Soma addiction. Rather than go to Sober Living, she insisted on going back to work immediately and attending an evening outpatient program. For the past five days, though, she's been missing from both. Now she is here.

"I thought she might do okay," I say. "She was a little self-willed, but she had a ton of resources."

"Opiates. You know what they need. It never takes if they go back too soon."

"Right."

"In any event, she's back. We have her keys. We got a urine from her and it came back dirty."

I spend five minutes with Debra, who cracks that she's back for the sequel. I do a quick exam, then go over the plan. She needs to detox and then go into Sober Living.

"If not, we're just wasting our time," I say. "My time. Your life."

She closes her eyes and groans.

"Got it."

By the time I get to the park, the sun is straining to come out from behind the gray clouds. I throw a Frisbee with the kids for a bit, and then sit down with the adults and discuss the disintegration of public schools, the cost of private education, and how we're all going to end up broke after paying for college. The conversation is easy, light—and depressing as hell when we get around to the high cost of medicine, the lack of old age care, and the strange diseases traveling around the globe.

"Isn't he fun?" says Susan, making fun of me to one of our friends.

"Is he always so upbeat?"

"You know Drew," she says. "The other day one of the boys had a deep cough. I called Drew, described the symptoms, and he said, 'It could be anthrax.' "

"I just wanted to grab her attention," I explain.

Then my attention is distracted by a guy sitting on a bench near the basketball court. I've already noticed him staring at me a few times, and now he's doing it again. I wonder whether I know him, and if so, from where. Then it comes to me. I excuse myself from the table, get up, and walk over to him. As I get closer, my memory becomes clearer. His hair is longer now, black dreads replacing the close-cropped look he had when he was in the unit. He's also cleaned up.

"Earle?" I say reaching out to shake his hand.

"Dr. Pinsky." He smiles.

I might as well be staring at a dead man. When he got on his bike and left the unit for the last time a few months earlier, I feared for Earle. I thought he was a sure bet to go back to using, that he'd end up another fatality. He had no inner self. He had no support system. His only way to cope, his only relationship, his only love, was drugs. He had nothing other than our feedback, and the experience of actually feeling better each day he spent in the unit.

"How are you?" I ask.

"Still sober," he says in a soft but clear voice.

"What happened to you?"

After leaving the unit, Earle explains, he went to Sober Living, where he met a woman who was also in recovery. When she transferred to another Sober facility across town, he found someone to arrange it so he could move there as well. Eventually he got a job in a homeless shelter. That led to a job with the Salvation Army, where, he says, he continues to work. He goes to twelve-step meetings at least twice and often three times a day. He also helps others get to meetings.

"I'm all about service," he says.

And in the process he is helping himself. He has gone beyond the terrible trauma of his past. He's no longer a victim whose life is about finding relief from constant pain and suffering. He has changed by thriving in a highly structured environment, where he has gotten the courage to trust and connect with other people. Those relationships have given him the chance he never had. He has a life.

"How'd you do it?" I ask.

"I don't know," he says.

This is the mystery of recovery. It is why so many patients attribute the change to God. I don't argue with them. I merely want an explanation of how they finally got it, and why, so I can give it to others.

"It's hard," says Earle. "Every day I wake up and have to get over my shit."

"How do you do that?" I ask.

"I just look at it," he says. "I talk about it in meetings. And I help other people get through their shit. That helps me."

"How does it help you?"

"It makes me feel good."

"What do you do when they don't listen? When they screw up?"

"I tell them to try again. I give them another chance. People are hard enough on themselves. My hand is always out for my brother."

After a few more minutes of catching up, I rejoin my family at the birthday party. The festivities are in full swing, with kids running around while the birthday boy swings a bat at a large piñata. I take a lemonade and mingle with the other parents, knowing my conversation with Earle has lifted my mood. Like so many of my patients, I am in awe of him and grateful for the gifts of insight and awareness he gives me in return.

Why do I love what I do? Besides the day-to-day medical challenges of treatment, I actually see patients decide to keep living. How can you fail to be inspired by the resiliency of human beings like Earle, by what they reveal about the resiliency of the human spirit? In so many areas of medicine, doctors and patients generally adapt to chronic illnesses, without necessarily getting better than they were before. But I see people get better than they ever thought they could be. And that is the rule, not the exception.

"Your next victim is in three-twenty-two," Alexi says, slapping a new chart in my hands.

It is afternoon, and I have returned from a heady lunch with Adam Carolla and our agent, at which we celebrated *Loveline*'s expansion into several new markets. Alexi has perked up since earlier this morning, when she complained about being bored by run-of-the-mill addicts and alcoholics following directions.

"You're happy," I say. "This can't be good."

"What a mess this one is." She smiles.

"Tell me."

"She is cocaine, Oxycontin, cannabis, Valium, and Klonopin."

"A total garbage bag," I say, mocking her.

"My kind of girl," Alexi chimes.

We enter the room, and immediately I see at the foot of the bed a sure-fire sign of trouble: a stuffed dog with long floppy ears. Alexi, having noticed where my eyes go, covers her mouth with her hand to stifle a laugh. I also note the usual collection of half-eaten candy bars on the night table. But wait. Look at that. The patient—I glance at the chart and see her name is Carol—has also put several framed pictures of herself as a child on the nightstand.

She's resting with her back against the wall, her knees pulled up to her chest, exposing rips in both legs of her blue jeans. She is knotted as tightly she can make herself. She looks miserable. And she sounds it, too.

"Are you going to give me something?" she asks. "I need something. My back is fucking killing me, and I want to jump out of my fucking skin."

I glance back at Alexi, who gives me a look that says, *I told you this was going to be fun.* I roll my eyes. *Let's get on with it.*

I proceed to her physical exam. Her heart and lungs are sound. Next I need to look at her head and neck. I ask her to open her mouth. And then I see the same thing I saw in Amber and so many other women with histories of sexual abuse. It is that peculiar pharyngeal relaxation, the submissive manner in which they put their head back and open their mouths. See it once, you'll never forget it.

"Did you have any trauma growing up?" I ask.

She looks surprised, her expression a mixture of *How dare you?* and *How do you know?* Mine, I hope, is passive, clinical, and empathetic, though inside I cringe. Confronting someone who has been afflicted by childhood abuse makes me feel something is dreadfully wrong. I believe everything, all of us, are interconnected in some way, our actions provoking reactions, and nothing beneficial results from this type of behavior. The opposite is true.

"I was four," she says, looking down at the blanket. "Routine stuff. My dad. He warned me against telling anyone. It was our secret. He was fucked up."

"Was he an addict?"

"Does the moon come out at night?"

"Pot? Coke? Alcohol?"

"All of that, and more," she says. "He was silly on pot. I actually have pleasant memories of that. But he was a mean asshole on coke. I remember times when my dad acted like a little boy, letting us ride him around like a horse, making funny faces, and letting us sit on his lap when he drove. But then one day when I didn't finish my oatmeal, he picked up the dining room table—the entire table—and threw it out the window, shattering the glass, the dishes, everything. If my mom said something, he'd smack her. Sometimes he hit all of us. Mostly we were scared shitless. But I learned to deal."

"How?"

"My dad left when I was eleven," she says, grabbing the stuffed dog at the end of the bed. "Life went on."

I wince when I think of the pain of the little girl traumatized at the hands of someone she loves and idealizes. When it's the father, it always affects her relationships.

"Do you have a boyfriend now?" I ask.

"I know what you're getting at," she says. "I've seen therapists."

"I was just asking if you have a boyfriend."

"Yeah, but I'll tell you what you want to know. All my relationships have been shit. I have trouble, okay? What do you expect? Actually, I know what you expect. But my question is this: What about me?"

"What do you mean?" I ask.

"If I answer your questions, are you going to give me something to make my back stop hurting? I have such goddamn pain, and you want to know if I'm dating anyone. What the—"

"I have to ask these questions," I say. "They help me understand you better. We just met. You're loaded. You're starting withdrawal. It helps if I know more about you."

"All right. My love life has been in the crapper. Can you call it a love life if there's no love? I had the dependent relationship, where I freaked out as soon as I started feeling close to the guy. I had relationships that were ruined because I convinced myself he was going to leave me, so I couldn't stand if he even left the room. And I've had times when I just fought and argued long enough to cause the breakup I convinced myself was going to happen anyway. I don't know. Just pick a guy and I screwed it up."

"Better you should push him away first?"

She looks away. "Whatever."

I know the sound of such indifference. It's the same helplessness I've seen in so many other patients, Amber included. If a girl like Carol pushes her boyfriend away first, then she feels like she's taking some measure of control, staving off the intolerable feeling of helplessness. A real connection with someone could expose her to the trauma of abandonment she first experienced with her father, and she can't handle that uncertainty.

I glance again at one of the photographs on Carol's nightstand. It shows her as a child of around five, playing outdoors with her older brother, who looks about seven. He is attempting to kiss her, and he looks secretly satisfied by his efforts to annoy her. She looks brilliant; her eyes sparkle with life. Laying on the bed in front of me is the broken remnant of that self, disconnected and addicted.

I don't want to imagine what happened to that little girl's lost innocence and the joy she should have experienced, but I can't help thinking about the terror, the fear, and the dismantling of her sense of life. Why aren't people protesting this kind of evil? We protest pollution of rivers and oceans, the cutting of tall trees, the loss of wilderness. We march against racism and hate crimes. We rail against films and TV series that are too violent or too sexy.

My stomach tightens at the thought that the little girl in the photographs is lost forever. She can never be recovered. My mind drifts to Amber. She is gone, too. She and Carol are similar, even down to physical resemblance. Carol may not be as stunning, but she is long and lithe and beautiful. She has large eyes and a small nose. Then I notice that the fingernails on one of her hands are polished pink. The other is natural.

"What's with the fingernails?" I ask.

"Oh, that," she says, comparing the two hands. "I got bored. Didn't finish. The story of my life."

Right about now is when I would usually start hoping for signs that Carol wants to cast me in the role of rescuer. In the past, I would have connected so strongly with the picture of the injured little girl that I would have taken her recovery on as a personal responsibility. I would have stepped in as a way of gratifying my own need to save her. But this time I simply stay with the reality of Carol as an adult. She is a woman of strength and resources. She has to learn to manage her feelings. My job is to help her on the road to acquiring those skills, without relying on primitive defenses like drug use or dissociation. In the face of the overwhelming stress of addiction and its consequences, she must find what she needs within herself.

Silence fills the room. I can sense something welling up within her. Here is where she expects me to step in to relieve her suffering, or attack or invade her with criticism. But I remain silent, as does Alexi in the background. This time the move is not mine. It is hers, and I am willing to wait.

About thirty seconds pass. Then I see tears flowing down Carol's cheeks. Soon she is sobbing hard.

"I am so ashamed," she says.

I reach for a handful of tissues from the box next to her pictures.

Finally, sensing that I might get a real answer, I ask, "Why are you here?"

"I am here," she says between sobs, "because I am such a fuckin' whore. I do this to myself."

My instinct is to swoop in and tell her that she's not not a whore, that she's not bad. Instead I keep quiet. I stay with her. I am there for her.

"I cheated on my boyfriend," she continues. "He wants to take my son away. I'm so fucked up. My life is so fucked up."

For a few minutes I try to imagine what it must be like to be Carol. The trauma she suffered as a child instilled the tendency to freeze and dissociate. This tends to make women like her perpetual victims. The usual story that follows involves rape during adolescence. She has continued to re-create the traumas over and over in her adult relationships for reasons she can't understand, and so she blames herself.

Suddenly her eyes lock onto mine. She looks angry, confused.

"Don't you guys ever say anything?" she asks. "Don't you want to tell me I'm fucked up?"

"Whatever you are, that's okay with us," I say calmly. "I'm just grateful you have come to us for help."

And I am.

Postscript

TO ANYONE WHO'S struggling with addiction, I pray that you find a way to connect. You must be fearless in evaluating your life, confronting reality, and casting off resentments, hurts, and fears. The only thing you can change is yourself, and only you can do that. But for that change to occur, you need an honest and trusting connection to others, not the cast members from all your past dramas, but caring people who have the wherewithal to help.

Every one of my patients enjoying successful recovery has discovered that the only way to get past pain, fear, and feelings of powerlessness or insignificance is by connecting with other people. They do it in meetings, with sponsors, with family and friends. Those new relationships are the building blocks of a new life. They provide strength and meaning, nourishment and definition. I advise you to look for opportunities to connect quietly and thoroughly and to participate in life.

And, finally, I hope that you'll all be able to accept a connection with something transcendent, something greater than yourself. Most people call this God. I don't care what you call it. Regardless of your beliefs, your brain on God can only help you to make healthier choices. It will force you to consider others before yourself. After all, we are not alone in this world. We share it with each other. And like Earle, do well by doing good. Always keep a hand out for your brother.

End Note

THE CASES I'VE written about are based on actual experiences, though I've carefully protected the identities of my patients. The last thing these people need is to feel exploited by someone they trust. Often I am the first person they have allowed themselves to trust since childhood. I have also exposed some raw and honest emotions on these pages, things many doctors would not dare reveal. In all honesty, I am not aware of many of these feelings when I'm in the presence of my patients, but they still exist, and writing these stories allowed me to explore this area in a way I never would in a therapeutic situation.

I think I have a fascinating job that offers lessons beyond the world of addicts and alcoholics. Life in the unit is real, raw, and bristling, like the severed electrical wire, with emotion. Most of the solutions the culture offers people today only intensify their problems. That doesn't happen in the unit. It's very nitty-gritty. But I believe that learning from the things that go on inside those walls can make all of us wiser, better, and healthier human beings. They have for me.

Acknowledgments

SUSAN, THANK YOU for standing by me through the crazy hours of my training and practice. My life would be so much less happy and meaningful without your love, support, and wisdom. I know that being my wife is not an easy job, especially in recent months when I had to forego family activities to "work on the book." I love you. Our children, Jordan, Douglas, and Paulina, remain the light of my life and will always be my greatest creations. I thank them for their support. Sometimes I think they pay the greatest price for my career—the time separated from their father. Thanks to my parents for their unyielding encouragement, for providing a safe and loving environment in which to grow, and for providing me with a world-class education.

Howard Lapides, Jackie Stern, and the staff at the Lapides Entertainment Group, thanks for your never-ending support and enthusiasm for taking my vague notions and turning them into projects of substance. It is because of your guidance and diligence that this book could become a reality. Peter Kusic, who was so much a part of your team, we shall all miss immensely. Jackie, I would not be able to make it through the labyrinth that is my life without you. Howard, thank you to Maria and the kids for the sacrifices they make so you can do the work you do. There have been too many moments where your guidance has been essential to list them all here. Your ability is truly amazing, but one piece of direction stands out in relation to this project. Specifically, thank you for introducing me to Tina Bennett at Janklow & Nesbit. Tina has been a champion of this project from the start. I feel so fortunate to have been shepherded through the process of development and execution by a woman of her ability and brilliance. Thank you, Tina, for your time, support, and essential contributions to the finished product.

A moment I shall never forget in the process of writing this book was my first meeting with Judith Regan, the publisher of ReganBooks. Tina had arranged a meeting between us at the Ivy Restaurant in Beverly Hills. After some small talk during which I complained about the lack of reality in the mass media, Judith challenged me to write twenty pages. She had heard what I thought was important for people to know and my passion for communicating it to them. That night she said words I will never forget, "Don't write what everyone thinks you should write. Write what is important to you. Write your book." I went home inspired, and twenty pages poured out of me. I e-mailed the story and she responded with, "This is your book, now keep writing." So I did, and it has been an absolute pleasure working with her and her organization since. I am doubly indebted to her for then introducing me to Todd Gold. Todd was able to take my loosely held together clinical observations and create a rich narrative arc. Todd has not only been a pleasure to work with and a skillful professional, but I now count him among my friends. Todd, thank you. Without your wizardry this book would never have taken form.

Calvert Morgan at ReganBooks is deserving of special mention. His advice was always precisely on the money. Thank you for being so responsive, supportive, and so damn right when there was more work to be done. Your editorial support was terrific. Valerie Allen has been working with me since the days of drdrew.com. Her consummate professionalism and ability have provided a platform from which to launch this project. Thank you, Valerie, for building the campaign to support this project so skillfully. Thanks to Greg Horangic and Sean Perry at the Endeavor Agency for their support and continued guidance. To Robert Eatman I give my sincerest gratitude for his amazing skill and dedication. A thanks to Anne Engold, the producer of Loveline for radio over these last many years. And Kevin Weatherly and Trip Reeb at KROQ Infinity Radio and Westwood One where I continue to broadcast Loveline five nights a week. Thank you to David Stanley and Scott Stone, who had the wisdom to take Loveline to television, and John Miller and Drew Tappan at MTV for making it a reality. Thanks to John Ferreter and Mark Itkin at the William Morris Agency for their years of hard work and support. Thank you, Jennifer Mendelson, for taking my rambling diatribes and turning them into great pieces for Frappa Stout at *USA Weekend,* to whom I am also grateful. To James Keppler and the Keppler Group, thank you for nurturing my abilities as a public speaker. Fred Silverman, thank you for bringing me into your life and enriching me with your wisdom. Thanks to Adam Carolla, with whom I have cohosted the show since 1995, for creating a vehicle that has allowed me to reach young people with important information. You may not always know it, but I am grateful for your remarkable ability.

Finally, thanks to the staff at Las Encinas Hospital. Those to whom I am most indebted are the dedicated staff that I work with every day who make my work possible, especially my charge nurse, Sasha Kusina; our clinical director, Michael Farinha, Psy.D.; and my physician partner, Barry Blum, M.D. These three form the foundation for characters that are represented in this book. Ultimately my greatest thanks goes to my patients, from whom I continue to learn about the human experience. They will forever remain a source of inspiration for me.

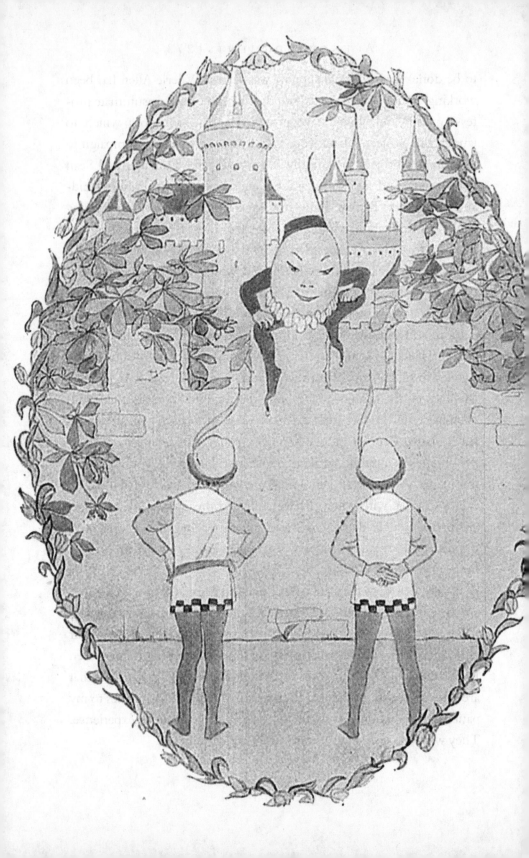

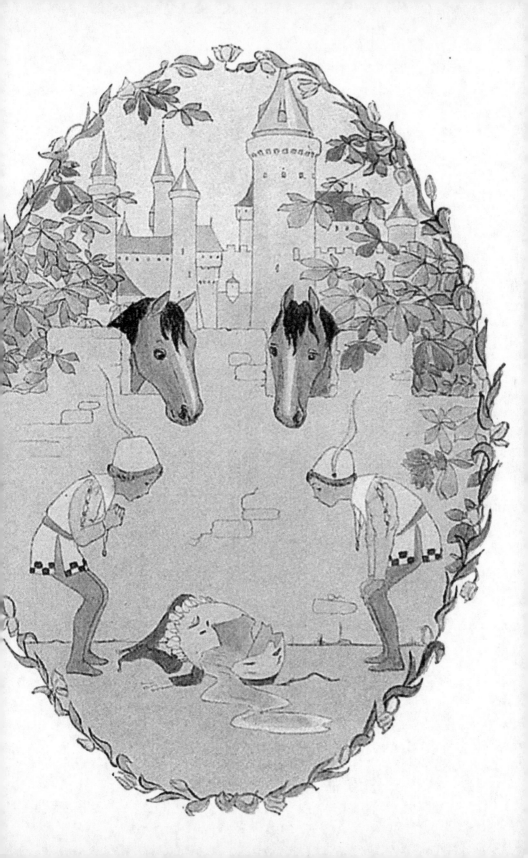